Reality of Hospital Administration

Reality of Hospital Administration

D Rambabu PhD (Hospital Admn)
General Manager
Department of Administration and Finance
Vijaya Group of Hospitals
Chennai, Tamil Nadu, India

Forewords
Mayil Vahanan Natarajan
Girdhar J Gyani

JAYPEE

JAYPEE BROTHERS MEDICAL PUBLISHERS
The Health Sciences Publisher
New Delhi | London

Jaypee Brothers Medical Publishers (P) Ltd

Headquarters
EMCA House, 23/23-B Ansari Road,
Daryaganj New Delhi 110 002, India
Landline: +91-11-23272143,
+91-11-23272703
+91-11-23282021, +91-11-23245672
e-mail: jaypee@jaypeebrothers.com

Corporate Office
4838/24, Ansari Road,
Daryaganj New Delhi 110 002, India
Phone: +91-11-43574357
Fax: +91-11-43574314
e-mail: jaypee@jaypeebrothers.com

Overseas Office
JP Medical Ltd.
83, Victoria Street, London
SW1H 0HW (UK)
Phone: +44-20 3170 8910
e-mail: info@jpmedpub.com

EU GPSR Authorised Representative
Logos Europe, 9 rue Nicolas Poussin
17000, La Rochelle, France
Phone: +33 (0) 6 67 93 73 78
e-mail: contact@logoseurope.eu

Website: www.jaypeebrothers.com
Website: www.jaypeedigital.com

Reality of Hospital Administration
First Edition: 2014
Reprint: 2026
ISBN: 978-93-5090-956-0
Printed at: Samrat Offset Pvt. Ltd.

The Tamil Nadu Dr. M.G.R. Medical University

Dr. Mayil Vahanan Natarajan
M.S. Orth. M.Ch Orth. (L'pool) Ph.D (Orth Onco) FRCS(Eng) D.Sc.
Vice-Chancellor

No. 69, Anna Salai, Guindy
Chennai-600 032. INDIA
Phone : 91-44-2235-3595
Fax : 91-44-2235-3698
E-mail : vc@tnmgrmu.ac.in
Web : www.tnmgrmu.ac.in

FOREWORD

There are a lot of books about hospital administration. This one titled *Reality of Hospital Administration* is special because of two reasons. First, the author Dr D Rambabu has condensed his vast administrative experience of running a tertiary care hospital network into this manual. Second, it is comprehensive and contemporary.

The book covers every topic not only for hospital administration but will also benefit the medical and MBA graduates.

I wish the author all success in his endeavor.

Mayil Vahanan Natarajan

ASSOCIATION OF HEALTHCARE PROVIDERS (INDIA)

... Educating & Advocating for Well Being of Common Man...

Dr. Girdhar J Gyani

PhD (Quality Management)

Director General

Ground Floor, Indian Medical Association House, Indraprastha Marg, New Delhi 110002, India
Ph: +91-11-23379651
Email: gyani@ahpi.in; Web: www.ahpi.in

FOREWORD

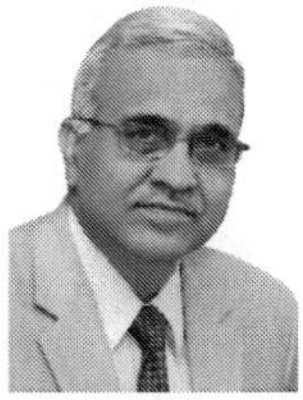

India produces the largest numbers of doctors, nurses and medical technicians. We consume the highest amount of US FDA approved drugs outside the USA and yet our healthcare reach is far from adequate. Our healthcare spending is less than 5% of GDP which is half of global average, the government share being 1.1%. The healthcare expenditure is estimated to be almost lowest in the world. There are serious challenges in terms of accessibility, affordability and above all quality (patient safety) of healthcare services. It is estimated that over 80% of national expenditure on healthcare was spent out of people's pocket, which is almost highest in the world. Life style related/non-communicable diseases such as cardiovascular, diabetes, oncology, etc. are proving to be serious threats.

The positive side is that private sector is coming forward to bridge the gap in demand and supply of healthcare services. Already this sector is contributing to the tune of 80% of healthcare expenditure and due to which we have some of the world class hospitals in the country. Healthcare industry is growing at very healthy rate. We need to apply modern management tools in this industry to improve efficiency (affordability) and effectiveness (patient safety). We need to quickly build capacity by way of educating and training doctors, nurses, and managers in the art of administering a hospital.

The book *Reality of Hospital Administration* by Dr D Rambabu, Chennai, is welcome addition to limited literature available in the country. It is amazing to find that he has succeeded in putting all possible elements in the book needed for quality governance of a hospital. He has used his vast hands-on experience in writing of this book and which will be of tremendous value to the budding managers in the art and science of managing a hospital. During launch of the NABH, way back in the year 2006, healthcare industry used to ask me for a single source of literature, which can help them in preparing for accreditation. While this book has one dedicated chapter on

NABH, some of the difficult subjects such as biomedical engineering, facility management, medical gases, operation theaters, medical records, functioning of various committees and the sensitive issues in day-to-day administration of hospitals, which is a challenging job for administrators have been extensively covered.

All in all, it is an excellent attempt by Dr Rambabu and I compliment him for bringing out such a useful material in the form of a book and which should prove to be helpful to the healthcare professionals and students undergoing medicine or hospital administration.

Girdhar J Gyani

Preface

With the increasing demand for hospitals, the healthcare industry has become one of the prime industries for capital investment in India. In 1980s, there were private clinics, small nursing homes, private hospitals, government hospitals, and public health centers. Now, the trend has changed, and the corporate hospitals started coming up with the state-of-the-art medical equipment and multispecialty services to the patients. Some of the government hospitals attached to the medical colleges are also providing medical facilities to the patients on payment at par with the corporate hospitals.

Secondly, the awareness of the medical treatment among the public has increased manifolds through the Internet, books, magazines, etc.

As there is an increase of healthcare providers, the ancillary services and industries are also growing. Some of them are nursing schools and colleges, paramedical courses in medical colleges, hospital administration courses, pharmaceutical companies, etc.

Because of increase in multispecialty hospitals, the demand for hospital administrators are also equally growing. It is a specialized course, which deals with the administration of hospitals. Since the hospitals are dealing with human lives, the administrators and the other medical, paramedical, and supportive staff require a special talent, training, competency, qualification and experience for running a hospital efficiently and effectively.

This book will give more practical knowledge to the readers about the functioning of the hospital, sensitive issues in hospitals, duties and responsibility of each and every category of employees in hospitals, patient rights and responsibilities, guidelines for accreditation, doctors do's and don'ts, and hospital systems and procedures, which are commonly followed.

I have collected some of the materials from the books, websites through Internet, journals, etc. Though I have taken proper care in collecting the material, there may be unintentional errors and inadvertent omissions. Hence, if there is any such unintentional errors, the reader is requested to excuse. I hope this book will be more useful for hospital administrators, students, and medical professionals.

D Rambabu

Acknowledgments

Anything to achieve in this world, one need to have many people who support his goals and objectives and this book is not an exemption. I am proud to say that my staff, from lower cadre to the Directors level, has given continuous encouragement to me during my 30 years of service in Vijaya Group of Hospitals, Chennai, Tamil Nadu, India, through which I have learnt a lot of things in hospital administration. First of all, I thank my management and staff. I thank my wife and children for their patience and support, without which it would be difficult to complete this book.

I thank doctors and staff who have helped me in proofreading and also my secretaries who have taken personal interest in converting manuscript into a computer document for easy correction.

My sincere thanks to Mr Jayanandan, Senior Editor who has taken a personal interest in recommending and forwarding the draft to the Chief Editor, New Delhi, for approval and also M/s Jaypee Brothers Medical Publishers (P) Ltd, Chennai, for their kind cooperation in bringing out the publication of this book.

Though I have written most of the chapters through my experience for more than three decades in hospital administration, some of the technical and medical information were collected from various websites and books. Since the sources were not noted properly, I express my gratitude to one and all who have helped me directly or indirectly to bring this book which gives real picture about the day-to-day administration of hospitals to the hospital administrators and MBA (hospital administration) students.

Contents

CHAPTER 1

Organization of Hospitals/ Healthcare Services

INTRODUCTION

Hospital organization is today an essential part of the medical care scheme. Owing to the increasing complexity of the medical sciences, it is very necessary for medical practioners and specialists to rely on sound hospital services. Furthermore, there is general agreement on the active role the modern hospital has to play in health and social welfare programs, and its influence on economic development of the country.

DEFINITION OF HOSPITAL

The hospital has been defined in Stedman's Medical Dictionary as:
"Hospital is an institution for the care, cure, and treatment of sick and wounded, for the study of diseases and for the training of doctors and nurses".

"Hospital is an institution for medical facility primarily intended, appropriately staffed, and equipped to provide diagnostic and therapeutic service in general medicine and surgery or in circumscribed field or fields of restorative medical care, together with bed-care, nursing care, and dietic service to the patients requiring such care and treatment" (Blakiston's New Gould Medical Dictionary Page 560).

"Hospital is an integral part of social and medical organization, the function of which is to provide for the population complete heath care, both curative and preventive, and whose outpatient services reach out to the family and its home environment, the hospital is also a center for the training of health worker and for biosocial research" (World Health Organization).

PROVIDERS OF HEALTHCARE SERVICES

The healthcare delivery system is vast and complex. There are a number of agencies or operators to provide healthcare facilities and services to the people. They may be broadly divided into:

1. Private agencies
2. Voluntary agencies
3. Government agencies.

1. *Private agencies* are the agencies where care is provided on the basis of fee-for services in a one-to-one relationship like private-practioners, nursing homes, etc.
2. *Voluntary agencies* are the traditional, nonofficial organizations established by groups of philanthropic and civic-minded individuals in response to the health and social needs within the community. They exist for unselfish and humanitarian purposes, with emphasis on 'service to the community' and as such, they play an essential role in the public health system in the country.

   Voluntary health agencies are supported by voluntary contributors, and hence are accountable to them. They offer free service and also involve in voluntary experimentation and research.
3. *Government agencies* are official health agencies operating at the local, state, federal and international levels. They are tax supported, their functions are mandated by law, and they emphasize health promotion and disease prevention. Official health agencies are accountable to the citizens and the government through an official appointed or elected to the board of the agency.

FUNCTIONS OF HOSPITAL

Hospitals have many functions to perform, which involve enhancement of health status, health promotion, prevention and treatment of injury and disease; the immediate and ongoing care and rehabilitation of patients. Other functions involve the education of health professionals, patients and community. All these activities must be conducted keeping the values and dignity of patients in mind.

A modern hospital is an institution which possesses adequate accommodation and well-qualified and experienced personnel to provide various services. These services are the cure of diseases, restoration of health and prevention from future illness to all the needy irrespective of their race, color, creed and socioeconomic background. Educational and training programs are also conducted in such institutions required for efficacious medical care and hospital service. Research to assist advancement of medical and hospital services programs in health education are some of the services that are taken up.

Thus, hospital is an institution provides healthcare in the modern world, by offering considerable benefits to the individual and the society at large. From the point of an individual point of view, the sick and injured person has accessibility to centralized medical knowledge and technology that render thorough and efficient treatment. A large number of professionally and technically skilled personnel apply their knowledge and skill with the help of sophisticated equipments and appliances to provide qualitative care to the patients. From the point of view of the society, hospitalization of a patient meant to cure him/her with the help of highly professional medical care, which is otherwise not possible at home.

CHANGING NEEDS OF HEALTHCARE SERVICES (HOSPITALS)

Indian healthcare service has evolved over the past six decades after independence. The role of private sector has played an important role in providing medical care services. Though public sector provisions dominated healthcare delivery in the first few decades, economic and political changes in the last few decades propelled the growth of private sector. Other factors that have aided the Indian healthcare delivery market are the changing consumer perception, increasing awareness about the quality of medical care, greater penetration of insurance, increase in purchasing power and the changing demographic structure. The recent innovations include focus on ambulatory and retail health care that are designed to focus on non communicable diseases. Inherent factors like improved efficiency, better quality, greater reliability and transparency have also aided tremendous changes in health care. With the incorporation of medical professionals under the Consumer Protection Act, 1986, there was an increased realization of the importance of quality in the provision of medical care services. With various initiatives of the Quality Council of India, efforts are underway to promote standardization of medical care services and thereby to enhance the quality of medical care that is provided.

PHILOSOPHY OF THE HOSPITAL

Philosophy is an abstract system of thought or belief that is concerned with the conduct of man's endeavors. As hospital organization is an essential part of medical care, it should have its own philosophy to deal with the day-to-day and future objectives. Philosophy is a statement of the value and beliefs that direct individual or groups in their attempts to achieve a purpose. Many hospitals in their definition of philosophy set their objectives and goals based on their vision, which may change with the needs of the society. Their philosophy also directs the organization in achieving their objectives and purposes. A purpose is a reason for an organization's existence; it is the 'why' of the organization.

However, every hospital needs to discuss critique and write down its philosophy in clear terms. No statement of philosophy of an institution is a permanent document; it may change according to the changing needs and circumstances of the society at large. The philosophy of the hospital is presented in its statement of definition.

CLASSIFICATION ACCORDING TO MANAGEMENT

Classification of hospitals based on the controlling board with change in times, hospitals fall under various categories based on their board of control. Some of them are as follows:

a. **Union Government/Government of India:** All the hospitals administered by the Government of India, e.g. hospital run by railways, military/defense, mining, etc. or public sector undertakings of the central government fall under this category.
b. **State governments:** All the hospitals administered by the State/Union territory, government authorities and public sector undertaking operated by the State/Union territories, including the police, prison, irrigation department, etc. fall under this category.
c. **Local bodies**: All the hospitals administered by local bodies, like Corporation, Municipality, Zilla Parishad, Panchayat like Corporation Maternity homes fall under this category.
d. **Autonomous bodies:** All the hospitals established under the special Act of Parliament State Legislation and funded by the central/state government/ Union territory fall under this category. AIIMS (New Delhi). PGI (Chandigarh) NIMHANS (Bengaluru), KMIO (Bengaluru) are some examples.
e. **Private bodies**: All the private hospitals owned by an individual, trusts or by a private organization, fall under this category. MAHE, Manipal (Manipal) hospital (Bengaluru), Hinduja hospital (Mumbai), and Vijaya hospitals (Chennai) are some examples.
f. **Voluntary agencies:** All the hospitals operated by a voluntary body/ a trust/a charitable society registered or recognized by the appropriate

authority under central/state government laws fall under this category. This includes hospitals run by missionary bodies and cooperatives like the CMC (Vellore).

CLASSIFICATION ACCORDING TO SYSTEM

According to systems of medicine hospitals can be classified as follows:

a. Allopathic hospitals
b. Ayurvedic hospitals
c. Homeopathic hospitals
d. Unani hospitals and hospitals of other systems of medicine.

LIST OF VARIOUS SPECIALTIES THAT EXIST IN A MULTISPECIALTY HOSPITAL

1. Anesthesiology
2. Biochemistry
3. Burns
4. Cardiology
5. Cardiothoracic surgery
6. Clinical apheresis
7. Cosmetic surgery
8. Dental surgery
9. Dermatology
10. Diabetology
11. Endocrinology
12. ENT
13. Gastroenterology
14. General surgery
15. Geriatrics
16. Gynecology
17. Hematology
18. Immunology
19. Internal medicine
20. Interventional radiology
21. Medical oncology
22. Microbiology
23. Microsurgery
24. Multiorgan transplant program
25. Neonatology

26. Nephrology
27. Neurosurgery
28. Neurology
29. Neuroradiology
30. Nuclear medicine
31. Obstetrics
32. Ophthalmology
33. Orthopedics
34. Pediatric surgery
35. Pediatrics
36. Physiotherapy
37. Plastic and cosmetic surgery
38. Psychiatry
39. Radiology
40. Respiratory medicine
41. Rheumatology
42. Serology
43. Sleep disorder laboratory
44. Surgical oncology
45. Transfusion medicine
46. Trauma and emergency
47. Urology
48. Vascular surgery.

CHAPTER 2

Classification of Healthcare Providers

CLINIC

In India, the term clinic refers to a place where a sick person gets doctor's consultancy and treatment as outdoor patient.

Though some of the specialty hospitals are running in the name of clinic like Mayo clinic in other countries, in India clinic has got a different definition.

NURSING HOMES

Nursing homes are one step above the clinics. These nursing homes are generally owned by an individual doctor or group of doctors. They admit patients suffering from general illness like fever, small injury, etc. and treat them as inpatients. But they do not admit patients with serious condition who may require intensive care treatment.

PRIMARY HEALTHCARE CENTER

Primary health care is provided by city and district hospitals and rural primary health centers. These hospitals provide treatment at free of cost. Primary care is focused on immunization, prevention of malnutrition, pregnancy, childbirth, postnatal care, and treatment of common illness.

VOLUNTARY HEALTHCARE CENTER

Voluntary health center are run with public or private funds for noncommercial basis. No individual trustee, or any member of the organization will get any benefit out of the profits of the organization. A board of trustees usually comprising of prominent members of the community retired high officials of the government. These voluntary health care centers charge fees from patients who can afford and very nominal fees from the economically backward patients. The main source of revenue is from the public and private donations, grants from the central or the state governments and also from philanthropic organizations.

PRIVATE HOSPITALS

Private hospitals are run by a doctor or group of doctors or nonmedical person as a proprietary concern or a firm. Compared to nursing homes, private hospitals provide larger medical services to inpatients and outpatients. These hospitals are run mainly on profit motive. The members of the firm or an individual who runs the hospital with private investment is the beneficiary of the profits of the firm or proprietary concern.

TRUST HOSPITAL

The hospital, which is run by a public charitable trust, is called trust hospital. The board of trustees appoints an administrator to look after the day-to-day functioning of the hospital. The board of trustees may be medical or non-medical persons. Trust can run nursing homes, small hospitals or multispecialty hospitals or even teaching hospitals. Most of the trust hospitals are run on no profit, no loss basis. Trust hospitals also charge the patients for the treatment, medicines, and facilities provided by the hospital. No part of the profit of the trust hospital goes to the benefit of any trustee or member of the trust. Though the Trust hospital is making profits, i.e. excess of income overexpenditure, the same will be utilized for the development of the hospital and expansion of the hospital.

CORPORATE HOSPITALS

The corporate hospitals and public limited companies are formed under the companies act. The capital amount for starting and running hospital is generated through issue of shares to shareholders. They follow strictly the company laws. For expansion of the hospital, the company will announce for public issue of its shares for an additional capital. The board of directors are answerable to their shareholders for their money invested in the company. These hospitals can be either general or multispecialty hospitals.

TEACHING HOSPITALS

A hospital to which a college is attached for medical/dental education is called teaching hospital. This hospital is for the care, cure and treatment of the sick and wounded for the study of diseases and for the training of doctors, nurses and other paramedical students. Teaching hospitals are run either with the government aid or by the private management.

ISOLATION HOSPITAL

These hospitals are located separately without being attached to the general hospitals. These hospitals are mainly for the care of patients suffering from infectious diseases requiring isolation of patients.

GOVERNMENT HOSPITALS OR ESI HOSPITALS

The government of every state is running hospitals in India. These hospitals are popularly known as government hospitals. Most of these hospitals are attached to medical/dental colleges. These hospitals are run mainly on government funds. Any sick person can be admitted himself in government hospital irrespective of her/his income position, status, etc. The entire treatment is given to the patient free of cost, even food by some hospitals. Paid wards or patients who can afford to pay for the facilities are also provided by some hospitals. ESI hospitals are run by the state government for the purpose of admitting patients who are the employees of private or public sector undertakings and, who pay ESI contribution to the government from their salaries.

The above classifications of hospitals are given based on the constitution, object, profit sharing, and charges to the patients.

CHAPTER 3

Hospital Administration

The success of any organization depends upon the effective and efficient administration and the clear and transparent policies of the organization. The policies of the organization should be easily understandable and known to each and everyone who is involved in the process of achieving the goals and the objectives of the organization. Formulating the hospital policies and implementing policies is a difficult task.

The administration in a hospital is divided into:

1. General administration
2. Medical administration
3. Finance and accounts
4. Personnel management.

GENERAL ADMINISTRATION

The following departments work under general administration:

1. Medical records
2. Hospital kitchen and dietary service
3. Laundry and hospital linen
4. Sanitary and house keeping
5. Security and fire fighting
6. Transport including ambulance service and parking
7. Building and engineering maintenance
8. Public relation office
9. Hospital communication
10. Electrical, plumbing, air condition department
11. Main reception and OPD

12. Liaison work with government departments
13. Hospital information system—computers, R and D.

MEDICAL ADMINISTRATION

The following departments work under the medical administration:

1. Duty medical officers
2. Nursing services
3. Paramedical services
4. Clinical investigation departments
5. CSSD
6. Operation theater
7. Wards maintenance
8. Imaging services
9. Medical gases
10. Patients grievances regarding treatment
11. Pharmacy and medical stores.

FINANCE AND ACCOUNTS

1. Billing department
2. Cash department
3. Accounts department
4. Finance budget department
5. Purchase department
6. Income tax, service tax, sales tax, excise duty
7. Insurance, TPA help desk
8. Corporate billing
9. General stores.

PERSONNEL MANAGEMENT

1. Personnel management
2. Establishment section
3. Human resource department
4. Employees grievances cell.

Though it is difficult to demark some of the departments under one particular administration, the above division of departments are given based on the broad activities of the department.

Some of the departments may function under one or two major administrations.

LEVELS OF MANAGEMENT

TOP MANAGEMENT

The board of directors and the managing director of the hospital, come under the top management. Mostly the policy decisions of the hospital are taken at this level. Plans for improving the hospital, starting new departments, expansion of the hospital, budget allocation are some of the matters which are dealt with at this level.

MIDDLE MANAGEMENT

The chief administrative officer/general manager—administration, medical director/chief medical officer, general manager—Finance and accounts, nursing superintendent comes under the level of middle level management. The officers in middle management act like a bridge between the top management and the lower management. They coordinate with the lower management staff to execute the plans and decisions taken by the top management.

LOWER MANAGEMENT

The staff other than the position mentioned above, are lower management staff. They work towards the implementation and execution of the policies framed by the top management under the guidance and supervision of the middle management officers.

DIFFERENCE BETWEEN ADMINISTRATION AND MANAGEMENT

NATURE OF WORK

Administration: It is concerned with the determination of the objectives and major policies of an organization.
Management: It puts into action, the policies laid down by the administration.

TYPE OF FUNCTIONS

Administration: It is a determinative function.
Management: It is an executive function.

SCOPE

Administration: It takes major decisions of an enterprise as a whole.
Management: It takes decisions within the framework set by the administration.

LEVEL OF AUTHORITY

Administration: It is a top level activity.
Management: It is a middle level activity.

NATURE OF STATUS

Administration: It consist of owners who invest capital and receive profit from enterprises.
Management: It is a group of management personnel who use their specialized knowledge to fulfill the objectives of an enterprise.

NATURE OF USAGE

Administration: It is popular with government, military, education and religious organizations.
Management: It is used in business enterprises.

DECISION MAKING

Administration: Its decisions are influenced by public opinion, government policies, social and religious factors.
Management: Its decisions are influenced by the opinion, and beliefs of the manager.

MAIN FUNCTION

Administration: Planning and organizing functions which are involved in it.
Management: Motivating and controlling functions which are involved in it.

ABILITIES

Administration: It needs administrative rather than technical abilities.
Management: It requires technical abilities.

KEY AREAS

Administration: Administration handles the business aspects such as finance.
Management: Management handles the employees.

SCOPE OF SERVICES

The scope of services of the hospital can be divided into four categories:
1. Administrative services
2. Medical services
3. Supportive services and
4. Round the clock services.

The main departments that come under the above mentioned services are:

Administrative service	*Medical service*	*Supportive service*
General administration	Various specialty services	Canteen
Patient grievances	Nursing care	Laundry
Personal and establishment	Investigation department	Transportation
Cash, billing	Inpatient treatment	Ambulance
Finance and accounts	Operation theater	Blood bank
Security services	Outpatient treatment	Physiotherapy
House-keeping department		CSSD
Main reception		
Insurance help desk	Others	Others
Others		

ROUND-THE-CLOCK SERVICES

1. Clinical laboratory
2. X-ray
3. MRI
4. CT Scan
5. Ultrasound in ICU
6. Ambulance service
7. Medical and surgical emergency services
8. Casualty
9. Trauma and accident emergency services
10. Operation theaters
11. Blood bank
12. Inpatient facilities
13. Pharmacy and others.

For better understanding of the patient, the hospital administration should display the list of major services that are not available in the hospital, besides the services offered. Proper board of directions should be fixed for the convenience of the patients. The outpatients should have an easy access to the investigation departments, billing and cash counters.

POINTS FOR EFFECTIVE ADMINISTRATION

1. The various departments functioning in the hospital for providing services to the patients have to be decentralized and the heads of departments have to be given importance and free hand to run their departments efficiently.
2. After decentralization of the departments, the management should delegate authority to the heads of the departments along with responsibility to take decisions in day-to-day administration for smooth functioning of the department. Both authority and responsibility go together. Without authority, responsibility cannot be felt and without responsibility, authority can not be given.
3. The management defines the clear policies of the hospital and also policies and procedures for each and every department.
4. The duties and responsibilities of the administrators, managers and each and every category of the employees working in the hospital should be defined clearly. Lack of clarity leads to confusion among the staff while performing their duties. If the responsibilities are not properly fixed they may expect others to take up their responsibilities which will badly reflect on patient care.
5. While fixing duties and responsibilities, the management should make ensure dual subordination of any employee. If any employee has to report to two masters or receives instructions from two officers the person may take advantage of the system and try to escape from the duties and responsibilities. It may also lead to misunderstanding between the two officers and disturb the smooth functioning of the department.
6. A true administrator never entertains gossip and back biting among his employees as it may effect productive work. In some hospitals the management keep itself informed of the happenings through specially appointed people. In such cases, the administrators should analyze and cross check the information before taking any drastic decisions. Information should be used only for the improvement of the hospital.
7. The management should fix the administrative hierarchy, and it should be informed to every employee of the hospital. All employees working in every department should know their position in the hierarchy and also the immediate reporting authority. Every employee should strictly

follow the protocols in receiving instructions and giving reports. Any deviation may lead to loss of interest among the heads of the department and senior staff. Since the hospital deals with patients, loss of interest among staff, lack of involvement in work, etc. may reflect on the patient care.

8. It is very important for the professionals and heads of the departments to involve in day today administration. They should be involved in taking decisions regarding the development of the hospital and improving the patient care and safety. Management should make them feel that they are part of the administration and also responsible for the development of the hospital.
9. Unbiased administration improves the morale the staff and also builds confidence and trust on management. Both promotions and punishment to the staff should be based on the records and good feedback. There should not be any personal favoritism where the patient care is involved. Most of the staff working in hospital relate to medical, paramedical, and technical areas directly involving in patient care.
10. A successful administrator should take quick and correct decisions. Since the hospital comes under emergency services and human lives are involved, important decisions like break down of generator, bursting of electrical cable, break down on life saving equipments, etc. cannot be postponed. The administrator or a responsible officer should be available round the clock for contact through telephone after office hours. Delayed decisions and hasty decisions may lead to complications later. Hence, timely decisions that lead to efficiency in carrying out work should be encouraged.
11. Attending on patients grievances is one of the important functions of the hospital. Since the hospital is a service industry and involved human lives, the hospital should have a separate department which deals with grievances of patients and their attendants. As it is already mentioned, the patients and their attendants will get irritated even for small issues. The difficult thing in life is to be a patient in a hospital and more difficult thing is to be an attendant of a patient. They may have health problems, food problems, etc. So, the person who deals with patients grievances should have the patience to listen their problems. Though some of the problems and issues are practically difficult to solve, the PRO should explain to the patients and attendants and convince them. Most of the issues can be solved by listening and answering their queries politely.

12. Every category of employee from housekeeping boy to the consultant is equally important to run a hospital successfully. All the employees contribute directly or indirectly their services for the care and treatment of patients. Maintenance of hygienic wards, bathrooms, safety of patients, prevention of hospital infection, etc. is possible only through the lower cadre employees, 'ayahs', paramedical staff and the nursing staff. House keeping boys, 'ayahs', male nurse aids (MNA) should not only clean and wash wards, toilets, but they also should attend to patients and also get involved in patient care. Hence, the administration should give importance to all cadres of employees working in a hospital for the smooth functioning of the hospital
13. The administrator should cultivate compassion towards humanity among the staff working in a hospital. Though the hospitals are run for a commercial purpose, the services are directly related to human lives. Hence, employees should help the patients, talk to them politely, console them when they are in depression and handle patients with care and compassion.

DUTIES AND RESPONSIBILITIES OF HOSPITAL ADMINISTRATOR

The hospital administrator is a person controlling all activities except those fields that fall under the category of medical care, finance and accounts of the hospital.

1. Though the administrator is not involved in medical administration, finance and accounts of the hospital, he should inform the CMO or financial advisor or accounts officer about his decisions, which affect the medical care of the patients and also related matters.
2. The administrator should make arrangements to conduct all the committee meetings, as per guidelines whether he is a member of that committee or not.
3. The administrator should allocate duties to all nonmedical staff as and the heads of the administration.
4. The administrator should delegate required power to the subordinates to achieve and fulfill the goals and objectives of the hospital.
5. The administrator should make sure that all the contracts are up-to-date and the contracts that are about to expire are renewed before the date of expiry.

6. The administrator should take quick and correct decisions since the lives of patients are involved. The administrator cannot delay the decisions regarding the replacement of life saving equipments, medicines, repairs and replacement of electrical generators, transformers, cables, etc.
7. The administrator should be on rounds everyday to supervise the departments and also to check the cleanliness of the hospital. His personal visits to the departments and wards will provide first hand information regarding the functioning of the various departments and also the maintenance of the hospital. This helps in taking proper decisions to improve the hospital services and rectify the problems exiting in day today maintenance.
8. The success of the hospital administration depends upon the effective allocation of duties and delegation of authority to subordinates. The administrator must decentralize and efficiently distribute the work rather than trying to do everything on his/her own. The hospital administrator should know the duties which can be allocated to others and which can not be allocated, but requires his/her attention.
9. The administrator should supervise all the departments to make sure that the hospital rules and regulations are followed strictly.
10. The administrator must make surprise visits/checks to the food cooked and served to patients, staff and visitors.
11. The administrator should see that all ambulances are quality of in running condition and are equipped as per the specification.
12. The administrator should maintain a record of all Insurance policies of the buildings, equipments, etc and see that the renewals are up to date.
13. Obtain all Licenses which are required to be obtained, as a statutory requirement to run the hospital and also renew on their due dates.
14. The administrator should get monthly reports from medical record officer and make sure that the case sheet of all discharged patients are deposited in the MRD on daily basis.
15. The administrator should develop a good and effective communication network at all times.
16. The administrator should review the hospital information system and report periodically and give suggestions to the top management to improve the services.

17. It is the duty of the hospital administrator to introduce the good systems in the hospital from the time of admission to discharge.
18. Manage biomedical waste management and its proper disposal, as per government guidelines.
19. The administrator should make sure that all the equipments and hospital furniture are in serviceable condition and dammed and condemned items should be disposed as per the hospital policy.
20. The administrator should ensure proper economic and should reuse any undue loss and pilferage to the organization.
21. The administrator is responsible for maintaining the discipline and decorum in the hospital.
22. The administrator should attend to the grievances of the patients and the staff.
23. The administrator should organize seminars by taking with the help of inside professionals or by inviting outside professionals.
24. The administrator should have a regular correspondence with corporate clients and insurance companies.
25. The administrator should conduct regular meetings with heads of the departments and get feedback to improve the services of the hospital
26. The administrator should keep the staff to aware of the policies of the hospital and also of their duties and responsibilities.
27. The following departments are supervised by the administrator:
    a. Personnel department (HRD)
    b. Medical records department (MRD)
    c. Hospital kitchen and dietary services
    d. Pharmacy
    e. Laundry and hospital linen
    f. Sanitary and housekeeping
    g. Security and fire fighting
    h. Transport and ambulance services
    i. General maintenance
    j. Public relations department.
28. The administrator also carries out the duties assigned by his top management.

DUTIES AND RESPONSIBILITIES OF MEDICAL SUPERINTENDENT/CHIEF MEDICAL OFFICER/MEDICAL DIRECTOR

The medical superintendent/chief medical officer/medical director is the overall incharge of the medical activities of the hospital.

1. She/he should ensure that all medical departments are working smoothly, efficiently with good economic sense.
2. She/he is responsible towards the nursing services of the hospital directly or through nursing superintendent/sister in-charge.
3. She/he should be aware of the medicals and paramedicals staff roaster and also help in preparing the roaster.
4. She/he should collect daily reports from the wards and for any deficiency solutions should be planned.
5. She/he make thorough personal inspection of the hospital every morning especially the patient care and overall working of the hospital.
6. She/he is responsible for the staff working directly under him.
7. She/he should ensure that the department of emergency/ICU is functioning with maximum efficiency.
8. She/he should provide adequate medical and para medical staff and equipments to all departments for their proper functioning.
9. She/he should control and maintain discipline among the medical staff.
10. She/he should ensure the patients to get the best possible care while they are in the hospital either as outpatients or inpatients.
11. She/he should monitor the turn around time/waiting time in OPD and investigation departments and she/he should try to reduce the patients waiting time to the extent possible.
12. Leave of all medical staff should be sanctioned by him/with his prior approval.
13. Personally investigate all complaints about the staff medical and paramedical and should report to the top management for appropriate action.
14. She/he should appoint duty medical officers or resident medical officers in the wards to look after the patients and to carry out the instructions of consultants.
15. See to that all purchases of medical equipments have his/her approval.
16. She/he should monitor the case-sheet of the patients and take proper action to rectify the deficiencies found by the medical record officer.
17. She/he should monitor the code blue team.

18. She/he should be responsible for dealing with all medicolegal issues.
19. She/he should assist the management for forming, coordinating and chairing of various committee meetings to improve the medical services in the hospital.
20. She/he should conduct clinical meetings periodically for duty medical officers as well as the consultants.
21. She/he should conduct training programs for junior doctors in various fields like BCLS and ACLS, code blue, CPR, etc.

CHAPTER 4

Important Components of Hospital

The given chapter brings out the important components of hospital without which the running of hospital is questionable: doctor, nurse, patient and medicine.

DOCTOR

Doctor is a medical graduate who treats mentally and physically sick people.

TYPES OF DOCTORS IN HOSPITAL

a. Resident medical officer or duty medical officer:
   A medical graduate is eligible to be resident medical officer and registered with Medical Council of India. An MBBS graduate is qualified to be a duty medical officer in allopathic hospitals. The doctor makes rounds in the wards and carries out the instruction given by the primary consultant or any other specialist. Day-to-day prognosis report is written in doctors note and discharge summary will be prepared for the patients at the time of discharge of the patient.
b. Registrar
   Senior medical graduates or postgraduates are appointed as registrars in hospitals. They work in wards, ICU, IMCU, CCU, etc. They are above duty medical officers and below the consultants.

They are assisted by medical officers. A registrar is guided by consultant, and after gaining enough experience is promoted to the position of consultant. A consultant can appoint a registrar to look after his patients, especially in casualty and ICU.

c. Consultants:
   In olden days, a single doctor used to handle patients with various diseases and sickness. But today many doctors prefer to specialize in one particular

area. So, a consultant is a medical postgraduate with specialization in particular field of medicine like neuro, general medicine, general surgery, cardiac, etc. Consultants also have diploma in superspecialty, in addition to their postgraduation. They take care of both inpatients and outpatients.

TYPES OF CONSULTANCY

1. Outpatient consultancy
2. Inpatient consultancy

Based on their functioning, consultants are categorized into four types;

a. Primary consultant:

Patients will be admitted under one specialist and they will take treatment from that consultant throughout the stay in the hospital. A primary Consultant is one who treats patients admitted under him and takes responsibility of coordinating with other consultants.

b. Referral consultant:

Based on the health complaints of patients, the primary or treating consultant refers patients to other specialist for his/her opinion. The treating doctor in additions to his/her treatment follows the instructions or the advice of the referral doctor. The referral doctor also visits patient as and when required.

c. Co-consultant

A patient with multiple problems receives treatment from different specialists. So, various specialists/consultants treat the patient with multiple health problems, by concentrating on their specialty area, but in co-ordination with other consultants. So each one of them is called co-consultant.

d. Changing primary consultant

When a patient is admitted under any consultant for treatment, the primary consultant will do the initial assessment and treat patients within the limits of his specialty. In case the patient shows further symptoms or diagnosed with different problem other than his specialty, after initial investigation, the patient is transferred to a particular specialist for further course of treatment. In such cases, the other consultant under whom the patient is transferred will become the primary consultant.

Factors that Contribute to the Success of a Consultant

The following factors should be kept in mind by a consultant for his/her carrier success

1. Availability
2. Accessibility
3. Affordability.

The consultants should be available in outpatients' department for consultancy of patients as per the scheduled time. She/he should also be available for consultancy of inpatients on call. Nonavailability of any particular consultant should be displayed in OPD for the convenience of patients.

A consultant may be available in the hospital but may not be able to accessible to the patients in outpatient department due to hospital procedures like hospital rounds, surgery, etc. In such situations the consultant may cause frustration among other patients. Though the doctors are available in the premises of the hospital, they are not accessible to outpatients. Such consultants cannot maintain good PR with patients.

Apart from the factors of availability and accessibility, affordability is very important. A patient should be able to afford the professional fee of the consultant. For example, if any superspecialist charges ₹ 500.00 to 1000.00 per visit as one time consultancy charge, patients may not mind to pay. But if the primary consultant visits patient one or two times in a day charges ₹ 500.00–1000.00 per visit towards his professional fees, patients may feel that they cannot afford to admit under such consultants. So, the affordability of patients regarding the medical treatment is also an important factor for the success of the consultants and the hospital.

DUTIES AND RESPONSIBILITIES OF RESIDENT MEDICAL OFFICER/DUTY MEDICAL OFFICER

RMO is one of the most responsible staff of the hospital

1. She/he should present all times of day and night on his shift duty.
2. At the end of his shift, he should not leave the ward till the other RMO takes over.
3. She/he is directly responsible to the consultants for professional work and they are administratively responsible to the hospital administration.
4. She/he is responsible for all the patients admitted in his ward for proper medical care.
5. Though a patient admitted under a consultant, the RMO is responsible for initial assessment till the consultant attends the patient.
6. She/he is responsible for carrying out the orders of the consultant.
7. He/she should ensure that all advised tests and procedures are carried out without delay.
8. On admission or in emergency, she/he will carry out necessary examination and history of the patient is noted so that the case-sheet of the patient is completed in all respects.
9. She/he should fill the required documents in case of medicolegal cases.

10. She/he should write the daily prognoses report in doctors note and sign the note.
11. She/he should inform to the treating consultant about the patient's condition and are action taken.
12. She/he will consult the specialists whenever required.
13. She/he himself should make rounds of all the patients in the ward at least twice a day and also whenever a patient requires.
14. She/he also accompany the consultants when they go on for rounds and ensure that all his/her orders are implemented.
15. She/he ensure that proper diet is given to the patient as per the advice of treating consultant.
16. Discharge summary of the patient has to be prepared by RMO. The discharge summary should be signed by both RMO and consultant.
17. She/he is responsible for nursing care being provided by the nursing staff.
18. She/he should explain to the patient about the precautions and medication to be taken after the discharge.
19. She/he should also get a feedback forms (regarding treatment) duly filled by the patient at the time of discharge and submit to the hospital management.
20. Whenever an infectious patient is discharged from the ward, she/he should monitor that the room is disinfected and fumigated immediately.

In addition to the above duties and responsibilities, the RMO who works in casualty or emergency ward has got additional duties as follows:

1. She/he has to perform the initial assessment of the patient as soon as he receives patient in casualty/emergency ward.
2. She/he should train the junior and paramedical staff in performing resuscitative measures.
3. She/he should also make sure that the initial resuscitation is prompt and adequate.
4. She/he should maintain emergency record as per the proforma provided by the hospital.
5. She/he should ensure that unauthorized abbreviations are not used in the case-sheet
6. She/he should pay particular attention to medico-legal cases so that accurate documentary evidence is available whenever demanded.

NURSE

A nurse is 'a person, male or female, trained to care for the sick, the injured, the old or the infirm'.

In olden days, nurse means a person who takes care of all types of patients. Though in the past, nurses were attending on people with different ailments; in modern times, the concept of specialization has entered the sphere of nurses also. After completion of nursing course a nurse receives special training in different specialties like IUC, operation theater, neuro, cardiology, pediatrics, NICU, PICU, casualty, etc.

Nursing profession is a divine profession where they serve all patients equally irrespective of caste, creed, religion, rich or poor, ensuring their safety and comfort by maintaining noble traditions of nursing profession, which includes complete dedication to patients' cure. A nurse should work in coordination with other departments.

Professional nurses are expected to demonstrate a certain degree of altruism, special attainment, self sacrifice and the right attitude in their dealings. Each nurse needs to understand the responsibilities and concerns that are integral to the nursing profession. Working with a team of health care professionals to provide care for patients in need, requires a discipline and internal and external composure that stays steady throughout the day.

The core values that are expected and appreciated in nurses are responsibility, honesty, integrity, belief in human dignity, patient equality, and the desire to prevent and alleviate suffering. A nurse's professionalism is judged based on personal behaviors, appearance, presentation, and so on.

1. **Non-Biased Care for Patients**

   Health care centers receives patients of all ages, sizes, colors, races and backgrounds. A nurse's job is to see a patient as a patient, and not focus on attributes that might be personally disliked. Showing any kind of prejudice will hinder the quality of patient care, and it also earn a bad reputation for the hospital. A truly professional nurse would ensure high standard, non-biased care for all patients.

2. **Integrity**

   Maintaining medical records for patients also needs a level of professionalism. Medical records are meant to be confidential. Nurses are trusted with a great deal of delicate information. The professional nurse should keep confidential matters confidential.

3. **Respect for Patients**

   Patients can be difficult to deal with, but a professional nurse cannot lose her temper. Its imperative to remember that the patient is in the hospital to receive care. A professional nurse is prepared to treat all patients with the utmost respect and dignity, no matter what the provocation.

4. **Attitude**

A nurse with a negative attitude can make things difficult for patients and staff alike. The nursing profession aims to help others than to focus on individual problems. A professional nurse will try to work well with others though she has got a negative attitude.

5. **Appearance**

People will always judge you by your appearance. When it comes to nursing, a nurse's appearance can either create confidence in the patient, or total mistrust. If a nurse walks in with unwashed or un groomed hair and dress, such a nurse would lose respect in the patient's eyes, the other staff, patients and their families will see you as, uncaring.

6. **Willingness to Help Others**

A professional nurse understands that everyone needs help now and then. Willingness to help is a part of a nurse's professional attitude that is most appreciated. A nurse who is willing to help other nurses, patients and patient's families is seen as someone who can be trusted, and who has a core of goodness. Goodness and caring are the ground values on which florence nightingale built the nursing profession.

7. **Team Work**

A professional nurse is a team worker; she understands that the entire hospital's staff has to work as a team to ensure ultimate patient care. a nurse who does not work well with the team can cause expensive hassles. In order to be a good team worker, a nurse must eliminate any 'self first' attitude. For example, when a hospital is full to capacity and all hands are required, a nurse cannot insist on taking vacation time off. This is the kind of attitude that shows a nurse is a team worker and not a selfish individual.

8. **Honesty**

Too much cannot be said about this vital quality in a real nursing professional. Honesty comes into place in several areas. For example, if a nurse has over medicated a patient by mistake and an error occurs, honesty in time will help save the patient. If you choose to lie and avoid taking the responsibility it only leads to cumulative issues.

9. **Responsibility**

A nurse has to take up a great deal of responsibility and must prove worthy of it. Everything from responsible patient care, to monitoring delicate equipment to which the patient is hooked, to responsible handling of medication. A professional nurse is one who takes this responsibility very seriously and understands the consequences of mistakes, accidental or otherwise.

10. Discipline

Last but not the least, let's talk about discipline. When taking care of patients round the clock, it would be so easy to just sit back in a chair and doze off. But if a nurse were to do that, medication schedules and patient monitoring will not happen on time, which means patient care is compromised. Secondly, nurses have to report for duty at the hour specified and relieve the previous nurse. Lack of discipline in any area will bring everything from mild annoyance, to downright chaos in a hospital.

It is the duty of every nurse to uphold the noble traditions of her profession and dedicate herself to the care of patients.

While maintaining the dignity and decorum of her profession, a nurse must at all times be cheerful, kind and courteous and sympathetic towards the patients and the attending relatives.

These qualities along with professional skill will win her the respect and coopcration of her patient.

DUTIES AND RESPONSIBILITIES OF A NURSE

1. Administrative duties:

   These duties deal with efficient and economic ward management though activities which are subsidiary, they cannot be divorced from the patient care.

2. Professional duties:

   General nursing care: These include care and attention to the patients in the interest of patients comforts and general wellbeing and maintenance of his/her physical health. A specialist not only attends to the patient with a particular disease but also include that are general in nature, which are common needed by all patients like dressing, hygiene, administering medicine, etc.

Technical nursing care: These include those tasks and activities concerned with the treatment and management of a particular illness disease with which a patient is suffers.

DUTIES AND RESPONSIBILITIES

The procedure laid down by the management for admission and discharge of patient must be followed strictly. The following are the important duties of a nurse.

1. Patient's case sheet should be prepared with all the particulars and details of patient at the time of admission.

2. A nurse should inform the reception about the bed number/room number of the new patient.
3. If any patient is transferred to the other bed it should be informed to the reception immediately.
4. Proper care in personal hygiene of patients like sponging, care of mouth, back, nails, etc. should be taken.
5. Other duties include servicing and removing of urine cans, bedpans.
6. Assistance and instructions to patients and their relatives to be given
7. Feeding of patients who cannot eat on their own must be done.
8. Accompanying with nursing superintendent and consultants for rounds is necessary.
9. Regarding policies/mediclaim and following standard procedures based on doctor's advice and recording the same in the case sheet is important.
10. Nurse should carry out canteen procedures based on doctor's advice.
11. Checking the emergency equipments by the side of the patient must be done.
12. Checking the flow or pressure of the oxygen as per standards should be done.
13. Periodical checking of stock of narcotic, sedation and other life saving drugs is essential.
14. Informing biomedical department in case of any breakdown of equipment in the ward is important.
15. Imparting health education to the patient and the relatives to prevent cross infection is necessary.
16. Collecting samples for investigation whenever required and getting the reports of all the tests done as per the advice of the treating doctor is important.
17. Documenting in the case-sheet about the patient condition, vital parameters, investigation reports, etc. is needed.
18. Informing the doctors about critical values of the patients for further treatment and carrying out the instructions given by the doctors is needed.
19. Escorting patients while transferring to and from the other wards/OT is necessary.
20. Supervision of cleanliness of the ward floor, bathrooms, sink, linen, proper placement of dustbins and bio medical wastage by housekeeping boys and ayahs should be done.
21. Handing over and taking over of the patient at the time of changeover of their duty hours.

22. Changing of IV fluid bottles on time.
23. Proper administration of cannular to the patient.
24. In obstetric cases special attentions should be given to care of breasts and perineum care, catheterization of female patient, baby care, assisting in breast feeding.
25. Periodical checking of linen and removal the torn sheets, pillow covers, etc.
26. Proper pre- and postoperative care should be taken in case of surgical patients.
27. Proper consent must be taken from the patient or nearest relative before surgery in the prescribed form in case of surgical patient.
28. Ensured that the additional advance has been paid for the surgery before sending the patient for surgery.
29. The emergency trolley or crash trolley should be maintained properly.
30. In case of emergency and if the medicine cannot be procured by the patients attendant, the same should be issued from crash trolley. It should be replaced by the attendant as soon as possible, to maintain the inventory.
31. Checking the blood group and other details before blood transfusion is mandatory.
32. Proper care should be taken, in case of bed ridden patients, to avoid bed sores.
33. Terminally ill patients should not be left alone.
34. Proper care should be taken while administering certain special drugs like dopamine, etc. and it should be done in presence of doctor on duty.
35. Teaching new staff about ward orientation and ward routine is important.
36. Sending the patients case-sheet to the billing section at the time of discharge.
37. At the time of discharge, all injections, medicines, etc. left over with the patient should be given back to the patient.
38. To see to that all chargeable tests or procedures and consumables are written in case sheet in charges sheet to enable billing staff to charge in the final bill.
39. Handing over the discharge summary to the patient at the time of discharge is necessary.
40. Whenever a patient with any communicable disease is discharged or a death takes place, the room should be thoroughly fumigated, disinfected and carbolized.
41. Any other duties related to nursing services.

Most of the duties and responsibilities mentioned above are common for staff nurse, nurse in-charge and nursing supervisor. Administrative responsibilities are more for nursing superintendent and general and technical duties and responsibilities will be more for staff nurse.

PERSONAL HYGIENE OF PATIENT: RESPONSIBILITY OF NURSING STAFF

1. As soon as she enters the ward, a nurse should wear PPE and hand washing and also wish the elders and the patients.
2. While handing over and taking over the patient, she must take care personal hygiene and check the patient head to foot, comb hair, eye and mouth care, etc.

PATIENT OR THE PERSON WITH ILLNESS

A patient is one who gets admitted in a hospital due to physical or mental illness. He seeks a hospital that is well known to cure him/her of the impending illness. Since hospital industry also thrives on the number of patients with major ailments seeking their services, it is necessary for the hospital to satisfy their customers, i.e. the patients. But there is a vast difference between the customer which a hospital receives and the 'customer' in general sense. In a hospital, the customer is forced to seek the services due to unavoidable circumstances, but elsewhere she/he has the deciding power in purchasing or rejecting the goods and services. But in a hospital a patient is totally under control and cannot do things with his purchasing power—costs that she/he incurs for illness. So, it is right to say that the patient in a hospital is an 'unwilling customer' with doubts and hesitation about the services she/he receives. Hence, it is necessary on the part of the hospital staff to build confidence in the patient by being gentle and compassionate even if the patient uses his/her temper due to physical and emotional problems. The patient/or the sick person may face inconvenience in the food she/he receives, constraints in his/her budget, face difficulty in transport besides her/his major health problem. So, the hospital staff should understand these problems of the patient, treat and attend to both outpatients and inpatients well, So that the customer is satisfied.

TYPES OF PATIENTS

1. Outpatients

A physically or mentally ill person who visits a consultant/a doctor in a clinic, nursing home, hospital for medical advice and treatment as an outdoor patient is called outpatient.

Outpatients may be a new patient or a review patient. If a patient comes first time to the hospital for medical consultancy, he will be registered as a new patient. Subsequently, if the patient comes for consultancy with the doctor he will be registered as review patient.

2. Inpatients

A person who is sick and required to be admitted in a hospital for treatment is called inpatient. A person can admit himself in a hospital as an inpatient for acute or chronic health problems. He will be admitted under a consultant for treatment. Then he will be referred to other specialist based on his health complaints by his consultant. One who treats him for his basic health problem is a primary consultant and others are referral doctors.

Inpatients again can be divided into following types based on the mode of payment.

a. Cash patients

They are like general patients who admit themselves in the hospital as inpatients for treatment and settle hospital bills by cash/cheque at the time of discharge, by the patient.

b. Patients referred by companies

As a part of welfare measure to the employees, most of the public sector undertakings and private companies are bearing the cost of treatment of their employees. These companies will have a tie up with private hospitals for treatment of their employees on credit basis. On entering into a mutual agreement by company with any multispecialty hospital, the company starts referring their employees to the empanelled hospital for treatment either as outpatients or inpatients as per the terms and conditions mentioned in the agreement. The empanelled hospital admits patients referred by the companies on submission of reference letters. The hospital provides the necessary treatment to patients and submits the bill to the companies for payment. If any disallowed items are in the bill, as per the agreement, the patient will pay the charges for the same at the time of discharge.

3. Patients claiming reimbursement of hospitalization charges from insurance companies

These patients are treated as cash paid patients. But some of the prescribed forms have to be filled by the hospital authorities and hand them over to the patients to submit to the insurance companies for claiming reimbursement of the hospital expenditure.

4. Patients referred by TPAs for cashless treatment

Of late many of the patients being admitted in private hospitals are insured patients, who holds insurance cards as the policy holders of insurance companies. These insurance companies will settle the hospital bills on behalf of their policy holders as per their eligibility, they are called "third party administrators" (TPAs).

These TPAs process the claims received from the hospitals and settle bills as per the eligibility of the cardholders or approved amount. Hospitals will enter into an agreement with TPAs. The percentage of patients admitting under cashless treatment has increased to 40–50% in multispecialty hospitals. Hospitals which have agreements with TPAs should have a separate department to guide patients and send required particulars to insurance companies.

The IT companies or industries are taking policy from one of the TPAs for their employees' medical claim.

The mediclaim cardholders can send pre-authorization letter to the insurance company and get approval for cashless treatment before getting admitted to a hospital for treatment, if not they must inform the agency within 24 hours from the time of admission in the hospital. TPA help desk sends a duly filled prescribed pre-authorization form and sends it to the company for approval.

The concern TPA verifies the particulars of patients', disease, number of days stay in the hospital, cost of treatment, doctors' fees, policy ID number, etc. and send its approval for cashless treatment as per the card holder's eligibility through fax or email to the hospital.

Most of the patients who have got Mediclaim Insurance Cards are under the impression that they can get admitted in any hospital and get treatment at free of cost by simply showing the card. But they are not eligible for cashless treatment unless or otherwise the approval comes from the insurance company. Hospitals are not obligatory to treat patients on cashless basis by mere showing the insurance ID cards by the patients, without approval for cash less treatment.

5. CGHS Patients

Employees working in central government offices like income tax department, excise department, etc. are eligible to take treatment in private hospitals, which are recognized by Central Government Employees Health Scheme. To get recognition for hospital by CGHS, the charges for various services provided by the hospital should be as per the approved rates of CGHS or if the hospital charges are approved by CGHS the Central Government

Employees are eligible for taking treatment in empanelled private hospitals. Hospital authorities send all the bills of patients covered under CGHS directly to the office of CGHS for payment. After verifications of bills, with their approved rates, the office of CGHS releases the payment to hospitals.

Some of the multispecialty hospitals are reluctant to apply for empanelment because the approved charges of CGHS are lower compared to the private corporate hospitals. Keeping this in view, CGHS has revised the charges for various procedures.

6. Arogya Sri or Government Schemes

In recent years the Government of Andhra Pradesh has started a new health scheme with an objective to provide medical treatment to maintain good health for the poor at free of cost with the introduction of "Arogya Sri Scheme". It has become very popular and received a lot of appreciations from the people of AP and also of other states.

Recently the Government of Tamil Nadu also has introduced a new scheme based on these lines. As per the scheme, any sick person of the State with a ration card can admit in any private hospital for treatment. He is eligible for treatment as per the rules of the scheme.

Private hospitals having agreement with the State government will treat patients admitted under the scheme and their hospital bills are sent to the health department or insurance company as per the agreement of payment. Patients admitted under this scheme need not pay the admissible charges to the hospital for the diseases mentioned in the agreement. Hospital will get payment directly from either the government or the insurance company.

7. Free Patients

Some of the trust hospitals and corporate hospitals enjoy certain benefits like income tax exemption on net income or customs duty exemption on medical equipments, etc. The statutory obligation on these hospitals is to treat 10% of inpatients at free of cost. They should maintain a register showing the names of the patients, address, doctors' names, hospital bill amount, etc. It should be available with the hospital authorities for any verification by government departments. Hospital allots some of its inpatients beds for free patients. These patients do not pay any amount towards treatment to Hospital.

The hospital authorities will decide the criteria for selecting patients for free treatment example like the annual income, ration card for low income group or certificate from a local body.

8. Hospital staff and their family members

Most of the private hospitals in India provide health facilities to their employees or their family members at a concessional charge or free of cost as a welfare measure to the staff. As per the policies fixed by the management, the staff is eligible for either outpatient or inpatient treatment at concessional rate or free of cost. The hospital bill amount is collected from the staff at the time of discharge deducts from their salary on monthly installments if the treatment is provided on concessional charge.

PATIENTS' RIGHTS

Every patient has the following rights:

1. Medical treatment

- Patient has the right to be treated with dignity, compassion and courtesy
- Patient can get appropriate treatment based on their clinical need regardless of culture, age, gender, religion or any social standing or sexual orientation
- Patient can get treated by a suitably qualified health professional
- Patient can receive emergency care whenever she/he needs/asks for it
- Patient can receive an outpatient department consultation at a mutually convenient time and to see the doctor within a reasonable time of the confirmed appointment giving scope for the doctors to attend medical emergencies and previous appointment patients
- Patient can receive medical advice and treatment which fully meets the currently accepted standards or care and quality

  (The currently accepted standards are those adopted by a responsible body of the profession in the light of accepted contemporary medical practice).
- Patient has the right to accept or refuse any medication, investigation or treatment as well as the right to information on the likely consequences of such a refusal
- Patient has the right to ask for clarification from the administration or a doctor of patient choice, in case a doctor refuses to continue the treatment
- Patient can ask for prescribed appropriate drugs and medicines
- Patients can ask for treatment with utmost dignity even at times of extreme critical illness.

2. Right to information

- Patient has the right to ask the names of the people treating and their professional capacity
- Patient has the right to ask for a clear description of their medical condition, with diagnosis, prognosis and of the treatment proposed including

investigations, procedures, surgeries, common risks, estimated costs, and appropriate alternatives, if any and to choose from them

- Patient has the right to be informed of the modification or change in the medical Management if any
- Patient has the right to receive a clear explanation regarding the services available in the hospital, how and where the patient can receive the same
- Patient has the right to know the names of any prescribed medication, and its normal actions and potential side effects given your condition
- Patient has the right to be kept informed of waiting time, delays and cancellations of various happenings.

3. Right to choose

- Patient has right to request for a second medical/surgical opinion
- Patient has the right to choose take part or not take part in medical research programs
- Patient has the right to choose the language in which inter personal communications can be made during their visit to the hospital.

4. Right to privacy

- To be in a clean, safe and secured environment as deemed medically appropriate during one's treatment while in the hospital.
- Patient has the right to privacy during consultant, treatment and hospitalization.

5. Right to complaint

- Patient has the right to make any legitimate complaints and have these complaints satisfactorily redressed in a reasonable period of time
- Patient has the right to make formal complaints either verbally or in writing to the patient relations officer
- The complaints are investigated and followed up by appropriate personnel
- Patient has the right to receive a substantive reply to any complaint within a reasonable period of time with an indication of any action that has been or will be taken.

PATIENT RESPONSIBILITIES

- Respect the rights and treat all healthcare workers and other patients and visitors with dignity
- Comply with all hospital policies and guidelines as informed or displayed
- Be available for any appointments made or notify the hospital as early as possible if they are unable to stick to the appointment

- Acknowledge that some other patients' medical condition may need urgent attention than theirs and accept that the doctor may need to attend them first. She/he should cooperate in such situations
- Take responsibility for her/his hospital bill
- Provide comprehensive and accurate details to the hospital about his past medical records and be complaint as regard to taking medication or following any other prescribed treatment
- Follow the prescribed and agreed treatment plan and carefully comply with the instructions given
- Accept responsibility for decisions he makes regarding the treatment
- Avoid taking medication independent of medical advice
- Avoid asking hospital to provide incorrect information, receipts or certificates
- Avoid wasting medical resources and time unnecessarily
- Accept, where applicable, adaptations to the environment to ensure a safe and secure stay in hospital with a full explanation from hospital staff
- Accept the measures taken by the hospital to ensure personal privacy and confidentiality of medical records
- Provide correct information regarding identity and financial status
- Strictly observe the hospitals' visitors policy as displayed to protect the environment
- Utilize the healthcare system appropriately and do not abuse it.

CHAPTER 5

Procedures in Hospital

ADMISSION OF A PATIENT

In case a OPD patient needs admission, the admission clerk or the receptionist should ask the patient about his/her preference to the class of accommodation. She/he should then inquire from the nurse about availability of bed of patient's choice. The reception should have upto date occupancy chart of the hospital so that admission process takes minimum possible time.

The admitting clerk writes patients' particulars on the case-sheet.

The helper should take the patient for admission in the concerned ward and handover all the papers to the in-charge nurse.

The nurse takes the patient to the room; orient him about the facilities available in the room and how to call the staff in case of any emergency/ any requirement. Then the nurse should inform the resident medical officer.

While completing admission formalities, the first and the most important job is to take the general consent of a patient for admission an authorized proforma. Signature from the patient, if he can sign (conscious) and his nearest relative, if the patient cannot sign (unconscious or illiterate) should be obtained in the prescribed form.

Writing of patient's particulars on each case sheet paper is compulsory.

If a patient carries any valuable items like cash or jewellery, she/he should be advised to keep those valuables in safe custody.

If an admission is done from OPD on emergency basis in an emergency ward the nurse should admit the patient immediately, start the treatment, stabilize the patient and then ask an attendant to approach reception/admission counter for completing the admission formalities along with the advance payment.

Here also consent is a must either from the patient or from any close relative before proceeding for further treatment.

The hospital staff should never insist on advance payment or completion of paper work in an emergency admission.

UNIQUE PATIENT IDENTIFICATION NUMBERS

In any hospital, the patient gets an ID number at the time of admission. This number is used as a reference number for treatment, surgical procedures, investigations, billing etc. This is called IP number, hospital ID number, etc. These numbers are allotted to patients on sequence of admissions from 1st January to 31st December every year or as per the policy of the hospital. If any patient is admitted for more number of times in a year, he will be allotted IP No for each and every admission. The case sheets are maintained for each and every admission. It is difficult for consultants to verify the patient's past records since different IP numbers are given for different admissions for same patient.

The QCI has suggested allotting one unique number for one patient at the time of first admission. The same number will be typed on all the bills in addition to his regular hospital IP number or ID number. This patient identity number (PIN) is a unique number.

How and Where to Allot the Unique Patients' ID

Whoever comes to the hospital for the first time for either outpatient or inpatient treatment he/she will be allotted a patient ID number (PIN) in the main/OP reception and register. This PIN in the computer with other particulars of the patient like name, address, age father's or husband or wife's name illness, consultant name, etc. will be used for retrieving patient data or for review.

Hospital should maintain a separate file for each and every patient.

Whenever a patient who has already registered, comes for either outpatient consultancy or inpatient treatment, his case sheet will be sent for review to the consultant's table in OP or to the ward in case of IP treatment. The treatment note of every patient will be entered in his case sheet. Though there are no. of IP numbers or HID (Hospital ID/inpatient number) numbers for one patient there will be only one UPIN (Unique Patient Identification Number).

In addition to OP treatment note the discharge summaries of patients irrespective of no. of discharges will be filled in their case sheets maintained as per Unique Patient Identification Number (UPIN).

These case sheets will be maintained in Medical Records Department (MRD). Immediately after discharge and the verification is over by the doctor the case sheet of a patient should come to MRD.

If UPIN is not known by the patient the receptionist, or person concerned can get the number through the computer data.

Proper system should be implemented to maintain unique patient identification numbers effectively. Of course it may cost more to the organisation towards infrastructure, establishment, etc.

ADMISSION THROUGH OUTPATIENT DEPARTMENT

If any sick person comes to the hospital for consultation with doctor as an outpatient he will register his name in OPD. After paying necessary registration fees he will be directed to the consultant chosen by him or based on his complaints.

After examining patients, the consultant:

a. Will prescribe medicines or
b. Advise for investigations or
c. Advise for admission.

The patient will be admitted in a hospital on the basis of an advice slip given by consultant. If the patient is not critically ill he will be admitted directly in the wards allotted to a particular consultant or in pool beds or specific wards.

Critically ill patients admitted in casualty will be shifted to the intensive care unit or to the wards after stabilization.

ADMISSION THROUGH REFERENCE

An ill person is advised by the general practitioner or a specialist for indoor treatment. The doctor refers the patient to the nearest hospital or to the hospital of patient's choice. As per the reference letter given by the treating doctors and based on the health condition, the patient is admitted either in casualty or in wards. If any specialist's name is mentioned in the reference letter, the patient is admitted under that specialists' care or the casualty medical officer decides the specialist under whose care the patient should be.

ADMISSION THOUGH REFERENCE LETTERS BY COMPANIES

The other category of patients admitted through reference is the employees of public sector undertakings or private companies. As per the agreement between the hospitals and these organizations, the medical officer of the companies refer their employees to hospitals for either outpatient or inpatient treatment.

In referral form the medical officer mentions the specialist's name, or the health problem of the patient. Accordingly the patient will be admitted in a hospital.

As per the terms mentioned in the referral form the patient is treated and the bills are sent to the company for payment under direct payment system (DPS). Charges disallowed by the company are collected from the patient at the time of discharge.

DIRECT ADMISSION

Patients who come to the hospital for emergency treatment are admitted directly in casualty. After screening or initial assessment by casualty medical officer, the patient is shifted to ICU or wards based on the condition of patient and kept under the care of Intensivist in ICU or the primary consultant in wards.

TRANSFER OF A PATIENT

A patient can be transferred from one hospital to the other or to a diagnostic centre for investigation or shifted to another ward within the hospital or to another department either for surgery or for investigation.

One of the important policies of hospital is transfer policy.

The transfer of patient means shifting patient from:

1. One ward to the other ward within the hospital
2. One hospital to the other hospital
3. One hospital to other hospital or diagnostic centers for any investigations or procedures, or
4. From the ward to the diagnostic departments or operation theaters for investigations or surgical procedures within the hospital.

FROM ONE WARD TO THE OTHER WARD

Within the hospital a critically ill patient is shifted to ICU. When the condition of the patient is stabilized she/he is moved especially when she/he does not require for support systems. Sometimes a patient is shifted based on a specialist's advice or on the request of the patient himself/herself.

a. From casualty/ward to ICU—when the patient is critically ill.
b. From casualty to wards—when the patient is stabilized.

c. From ICU to wards—when the patient does not require life-supporting equipments.
d. From ward to ward—on the patient's choice or specialist's advise.

FROM ONE HOSPITAL TO OTHER HOSPITAL

Usually shifting of the patient from one hospital to other hospital occurs in the following situations:

a. Due to non-availability of speciality treatment.
b. Due to non-availability of rooms or beds or ventilators in case of emergency situation. In emergencies after preliminary screening by the consultant, treatment is given till the condition of the patient becomes stable. This is important because, critically ill patients should not be refused admission into hospital on any grounds. When the situation is favourable for transfer, the patient is shifted to a hospital of his/her choice. Sometimes an unwilling patient needs to be convinced by the chief medical officer or staff on duty for such transfer, as treatment from hospital is sought by patients because of the Trust they have in it.

FROM WARD TO THE DIAGNOSTIC DEPARTMENT

Sometimes a patient is shifted to a diagnostic centre for specialized investigations. In such situations where some of the diagnostic facilities or procedures are not available in the hospital, patients who requires those test will be transferred to the out side diagnostic centers or hospitals for such a test and the patients come back to the main hospital after the completion of tests or procedures.

When patients require investigations and surgical procedures they are taken to respective departments for tests or procedures within the hospital premises. After completion of those tests and procedures they are brought back to their wards.

To transfer or shift a patient from his bed to other places as mentioned above, the hospital should have a clear-cut policy for transfer. The policy should reveal:

a. How the patient is transferred or shifted.
b. Specification about those who accompany the (patient staff nurse, boy, paramedical, doctor, etc).
c Safety of the patient.
d. The staff must carry a case sheet along with the patient and must follow the procedures for handing over and taking over of the patient.

DISCHARGE OF A PATIENT

Every hospital should have a clear cut policy and procedure for the discharge of the inpatients. This policy is to ensure satisfaction of the patient by avoiding delay in discharge. Most of the patients immediatly wanted to be discharged, but the discharge procedure takes four to six hours of time after the treating doctor gives consent for discharge. Usually the nursing officer goes on rounds with the consultant for two to three hours and after their return they prepare the discharge report. So, it is better to avoid unpleasant situations with complaining patients by having the discharge plan a day in advance. Coordination among various departments ensures the smooth discharge of a patient. The duty doctor should prepare discharge summaries as per the details in case-sheet, a copy of which is given to the patient at the time of discharge.

REGULAR DISCHARGE

- The patient can only be discharged on instructions of the treating consultant
- The patient is to be informed about the discharge only after the discharge is planned
- The Nursing staff will arrange for the doctor's summary report and send it to the discharge summary department for getting it typed
- Prescription is given to the patient attender to purchase the follow-up medicines
- Nursing staff files the case sheet according to the checklist given on the discharge file
- Nursing in-charge checks the file and counter signs on the file
- Pharmacy card is filed in the discharge file by the nursing in-charge/ nursing staff and send through the ward boy for verification to billing department
- Discharge slip is given to the attender to pay the dues and clear the bill
- Attender comes back with clearance slip from billing section/cash counter and handover to duty nurse
- The In-charge nurse should check the file's charge slip. If any procedure is left, she should add in the charge slip and send the complete file for billing. Meanwhile, the resident doctor has to prepare the discharge slip with all instructions, medicines, etc.
- If any medicine is left over and is not required after discharge, it should be handed over to the patient for further disposal in a manner he deems fit
- Once the patient makes the payment, charge nurse should check the room for the all hospital equipments, TV, linen, etc.

- The duty nurse should explain the follow-up medicines, diet, physiotherapy if any, and when the patient must come for review
- The duty nurse should handover the discharge summary and all the reports after obtaining signature
- The paramedical staff helps the patient in dressing and the ward boy takes the patient out in the wheel chair to the vehicle if required
- The completed case-sheet is checked and then is dispatched to the MRD staff from where acknowledgement is be collected.

DISCHARGE AT REQUEST

Sometimes when the patient becomes stable and he wants to get discharged from the hospital before the advice of the treating doctor it will be recorded as “Discharge at request’.

Patient or attendant has to sign in “Discharge at request form” and follow the discharge procedure as normal discharge. The hospital is not responsible for any consequences arisen due to discharge of the patients at request.

DISCHARGE AGAINST MEDICAL ADVICE

Some of the patients might want to get discharged against medical advice or attendants might want to discharge his patients against medical advice.

The reasons for discharge against medical advice are:

1. Not able to meet the hospital expenditure
2. For sentimental reasons on terminally ill patients
3. Not happy with the treatment
4. To admit in nearby hospital for convenience.

Patients or attendants who want to be discharge against medical advice shall be explained about the consequences of their discharge and a written statement should be taken from the patient/attendant in case of unconscious patients.

After obtaining signature in a prescribed ‘Discharge against Medical Advice’ form, the patient is discharged as per the discharge procedures.

ABSCONDED PATIENTS

If a patient leaves the Hospital without any intimation to the ward staff or without the doctor’s advice and regular discharge procedures, it should be recorded on patient’s medical record as was ‘absconded’.

The matter has to be informed to the hospital authorities and to the local police. This has to be done after searching the patient around the area of his stay. If she/he is not found it should be informed to the nursing superintendent, medical superintendent, treating doctor, hospital authorities, security office, etc.

After confirming from the family members that patient has not gone home, it should be informed to the local police authorities. The following details should be documented in the patient case-sheet:

1. Time of absence when it was first noticed, steps taken to locate the patient
2. Condition of the patient prior to leaving the hospital
3. Family members' declaration and signature
4. Copy of the intimation letter sent to the police
5. Intimation to the hospital authorities and the note of the treating doctors with their signature
6. However, the matter should be discussed with the safety and risk management committee.

CHAPTER 6

Outpatient Department

Outpatient department (OPD) is one of the most important department in hospital. OPD is the place where all the specialists are available for outpatients' consultation as per the timings allotted to them. In most of the hospitals OP department will function from 8 am to 8 pm. The patients will assess the quality of care in hospital through the healthcare services provided in OP department. The outpatient care should be available round the clock in hospital either through casuality for walk in patients or through emergency department for sick patients.

EFFECTIVE RUNNING OF OUTPATIENT DEPARTMENT

1. OPD should be at the entrance of the hospital
2. OPD should have easy access to out patients
3. Proper facilities should be provided in OPD for wheel chair patients and vulnerable patients
4. Basic diagnostic units should be nearer to OPD
5. All new patients who come for OP consultation with various specialist consultants should be registered in OPD reception
6. All review patients also must be registered
7. The secretaries of doctors or OPD receptionist should send patients to doctor's consulting rooms as per the registration number
8. Crowding of OPD should be avoided
9. All specialists should available in OPD for consultation of patients as per their scheduled timings
10. All consultants names and their specialty should be displayed in OPD prominently

11. If any consultant is not attending OPD it also should be mentioned in OPD either near the reception or his consulting room, patients who have taken prior appointment with specific consultant should also be informed
12. Toilets for normal walking patients and special toilets for vulnerable patients should be provided in OPD
13. The medical store or pharmacy should be available near to OPD
14. The medicines mentioned in Drug Formulary of the hospital which are regularly prescribed by various specialists should be available in pharmacy
15. The patients OP records must be maintained in OPD for review purpose
16. Collection of suggestions and feedback forms are very much helpful for improving various healthcare services in OPD
17. Wheel chair, patient shifting trolleys, oxygen pipeline or cylinder must be available in OPD for emergency
18. Efficient security system increases the confidence levels of the patient.
19. The important key indicator for OPD receptionists is to minimize the waiting period of patients.

DUTIES AND RESPONSIBILITIES OF OUTPATIENT DEPARTMENT RECEPTIONIST

- When a patient approaches OPD, She/he should be immediately attended by the staff in OPD reception, either for enquiring or for registration
- The patient's details should be collected and entered in a OPD register or computer
- Cash should be collected for registration and professional fees for doctors and issued a card with required details fill in, before directing patients to see the consultant
- During OPD timings as per the policy of the hospital no patient should be refused for registration
- Once the patient has registered in OPD it stands valid for a particular period as decided by the management
- Even if patients wish to see one or more consultants, the patient need not pay the registration charges within the stipulated period. Only the professional fees for doctors is collected
- Separate file for each and every patient should be maintained in OPD according to their registration numbers

- The clinical history of patients is to be entered in the file by the consultant along with the investigation referred and reports have to be filed in the patient's record file
- Whenever a review patient comes for consultation with doctors the file of such patient is to be taken from the record room and given it to the patients for doctors' reference and updating
- Preference should be given to vulnerable patients like very sick, old, physically challenged, children, etc.
- If the appointments with doctors are centralized, the OPD receptionist should maintain proper records for all appointments of consultants. It should be informed to the consultants
- In case of non-availability of any consultant on a particular day OPD receptionist should put a board in the OPD about the absence and also intimate all the patients through phone, who have taken prior appointments
- Unwanted persons wondering in OPD should be strictly observed and restricted
- OPD and toilets in OPD should be kept clean
- Required reports should be prepared and submitted to the administrators periodically
- The main key indication for OPD receptionist is to reduce the waiting time of patient.

CHAPTER 7

Diagnostic Departments: Central Billing

Patients who come to the hospital for OP or IP treatment are referred to different departments for various tests by the consultants. Mostly the line of treatment depends on the medical reports given by various diagnostic departments like clinical laboratory, radiology, CT, MRI, nuclear scan, ultrasound, ECG, etc. Among these departments clinical laboratory plays an important role as every patient has to undergo the laboratory test as a basic investigation before starting an active treatment.

Patients undergo various tests one after the other as per the advice of the doctors. It is advisable to have all the investigation facilities/departments are available/located at one place for the convenience of the patient.

There should be a central OP billing section for all investigations, instead of having different billing for different test. The cash counter should be adjacent to the billing section to enable the patients to make payments immediately without making them to run pillar to post. There can be two cash counters. One cash counter is for main transaction like IP billing receipts, payment for day-to-day cash expenditure, miscellaneous receipts, etc. and an another cash counter should be only for outpatient collections for investigations, registrations, miscellaneous receipts like canteen, physiotherapy charges, etc.

Waiting hall with rest rooms for patients to sit and wait for their turn to go for different tests should be provided. Separate toilet for vulnerable patients should be provided with the facility of going inside the toilet with wheel-chair and the grab bars should be provided inside the toilets.

BILLING PROCEDURES

GENERAL

- Patient goes to the central OP billing department with requisition slip given by the doctors for various tests
- The staff in OP billing counter will prepare a bill for tests prescribed by the doctors and raise a slip showing patient name, bill number and bill amount
- Patient has to collect the slip number and confirm the bill number and bill amount
- After receiving the cash, the cashier will raise the bill from the computer and put the paid seal on the bill
- After confirming that the patient has paid the bill amount for the test, the concern department will do the test
- Patients have to collect reports from the reports counter as per the time mentioned in the bill or oral information.

The staff in central OP billing counter should direct patients properly. If there is any order of preference for test it should be informed to the patients. For example, if any patient has been asked by the consultant to undergo lab test, urine tests and abdominal ultrasound test. Generally patients go first to laboratory, give the blood and urine for test and then go to ultrasound department for abdominal test. For abdominal test, the bladder of patient should be full, otherwise plenty of water has to be taken and wait till the bladder is full. As she/he has already given urine for test his bladder becomes empty and he will be asked to wait for a minimum of one hour to two hours till his bladder is full. One simple direction that he should take abdominal ultrasound first before passing urine, she/he will save lots of time.

The advantages of raising a slip in the OP billing counter and bill in the cash counter after payment is that it can avoid the number of nonpayment of bills by the patient.

FUNCTIONS OF THE DEPARTMENT

SPECIFIC PROCEDURES

1. The investigation departments should work round the clock or during specific timings depending on the need.
2. The outpatient should go to the department personally with an appropriate requisitions and payment slip.
3. The technician on duty should attend on patient.

4. The in-charge of the department should monitor the waiting time of patients and should make possible efforts to reduce the waiting time.
5. There should be a fool proof mechanism of labeling the specimens, X-ray films, etc. while testing and writing reports in the register.
6. Staff working in laboratory should take utmost care not to mix up the specimens and marking on the test tubes and vials should be done with great care.
7. While disposing the waste, one should follow the norms of "disposal of biomedical waste."
8. The test reports should be written in the department register. It is useful for future reference and will be available on demand for duplicate reports.
9. Preference should be given to sick and vulnerable patients.
10. The in-charge of the department and other technicians should maintain the equipments in working condition and the higher authorities should be informed if any defect is noticed.
11. The delivery of the reports should be planned by the in-charge in such a way so as to reach the ward before the consultant's rounds.
12. The patient should be informed about the day and time to collect his/her report.
13. There should not be any unnecessary delay in providing reports to outpatient and inpatients as it delays their treatment.
14. There should be a coordination between the technician and the receptionist to serve the patients better.
15. Every department in-charge should calculate the actual cost of each test as a part of financial analysis, and it should be informed to the administrators every year as this helps in running the department economically and efficiently.
16. The departments should be kept clean and all the staff should follow the hand wash technique wherever applicable.
17. Proper care should be taken while washing glassware.
18. In radiology department, radiation safety measures should be taken.
19. While administering contrast material on patient, it should be informed to the patient and consent should be taken.
20. The statutory licenses/permissions wherever is required should be obtained and kept a copy of it in the department.
21. The technicians should wear personal protective equipment (PPE) as applicable to their department.
22. The department should keep the required chemicals and X-ray films.

CHAPTER 8

Pharmacy

It is a place where the preparation, dispensing, distribution and charging for pharmaceutical drugs to inpatients as well as outpatients.

In addition to thc policies regarding various procedures in pharmacy like, preparation, storage, issue, inventory of drugs, adverse reaction, medication recall, high risk medication, etc. the administration should have clear policies regarding the services to the patients.

EFFECTIVE PHARMACY SERVICES

1. It should have a good system of billing.
2. All medicines mentioned in a drug formulary should be available in a pharmacy.
3. It should provide separate billing counter for small prescription and cash bills.
4. Cash counters should be available next to the billing counter.
5. Token issue system can improve the discipline in the counter.
6. A qualified pharmacist should be appointed.
7. Periodical checking of expired drugs is necessary.
8. Proper care is required in the issue of narcotic drugs.
9. There should be proper control on purchases, issues and inventory.
10. Right billing as per doctors' prescription.
11. Right issue of medicines as per the bill.
12. Proper care in the issue of look alike and sound alike medicines should be taken.
13. More staff in billing and issue counters during peak hours of the pharmacy should be provided.
14. Adequate staff should be recruited.

15. Return of medicines should be accounted properly.
16. Proper storage facility should be provided to keep certain special drugs under specified temperature.
17. Clear policy is required for condemnation of expired drugs, contaminated drugs broken vials, shortage of drugs or excess stock, etc. and it should be documented properly.

One of the important key indicators for an efficient pharmacy is reducing waiting period and issue of the right medicine to the right patient.

RIGHT BILLING AND RIGHT ISSUES

Since pharmacy deals with life saving drugs, the staff working in the pharmacy should be alert and cautious while making bills and issuing medicines.

The billing clerk should have knowledge of medicines and he should be trained in computer operation. He should also have one more talent of reading and understanding the prescriptions written by various consultants or nursing staff. He should select the correct medicine written in prescription while making the bill.

The sales person in the pharmacy counter issues medicines for the patient based on prescription/bill. If he issues medicines based on the bill he has to verify and confirm whether the bill has been prepared correctly as per the prescription. He should be more careful while issuing look alike and sound alike drugs (example: Ketamin-Ketinov). These medicines should be kept separately in the rack in pharmacy.

RETURN OF MEDICINES

A hospital should have a clear cut policy regarding the return of medicines by the patients. If there is no effective system of taking back the medicines which are unused in the wards for patients, it will lead to loss to the hospital.

If return of medicines is not accepted it would be difficult to convince the patients. The patients may argue that they are not responsible for unused medicines as the medicines are bought on the advice/prescription of doctors. If doctors change the prescription due to so many reasons like drugs which did not suit the patients, change of line of treatment, drug that is not effective, drug allergy, etc. patient may not be willing to bear the cost of unused medicines. He shall certainly return the medicines to the pharmacy. For no fault of the patients, hospital cannot expect patients to ignore the unused medicines especially which are very costly.

Hence, the hospital should have a good system of controlling the return of medicines. To reduce the number of return of medicines the ward nurse can write a prescription for medicines required for two to three days for one patient instead of prescribing for a week.

Secondly, the pharmacy can take back the medicines which are not opened or cut the strips of tablets where the name of the drug is available.

Proper entries should be made in computers for all medicines returned by the patients to have a better control on inventory.

SUBSTORES

Every multispecialty hospital should have substores adjacent to the pharmacy counter or in the same building except small nursing homes, clinics where it is not economical to maintain stock in substores as well as sales counter. The purpose of maintaining substores is mainly to maintain buffer stock in the substores. As soon as the counter stock is exhausted, the medicines will be issued from substores to the counter. The substores will take care of the counter till the supplies are made by the parties on orders. This will reduce the number of nonavailable medicines.

If a counter gets stock from central purchase department or direct supplies to the counter by the suppliers, there will be very poor control on stock. The pharmacist may not know the stock position till the last tablet is issued.

Secondly, lots of medicines will be dumped in the counter, and then, it is difficult to maintain inventory.

The advantages of substores is:

a. It will reduce the inventory in the counter.
b. It will have better control on inventory.
c. It will reduce the number of non available medicines.
d. It will reduce pilferage and misuse of medicines.
e. More accountability can be fixed on counter staff.
f. Reorder level of medicines that can be maintained effectively.

Re-order level can be fixed based on the movement analysis of each and every drug. There are: (1) Fast moving drugs, (2) slow moving drugs, and (3) rare moving but life saving drugs. While fixing re-order level, it should be done by keeping in view the quantity required for number of days (one week or ten days) of a particular drug. If the reorder quantity is more there will be excess stock. If it is less there will be shortage of stock. Hence continuous monitoring is required on the movement of drugs and the reorder levels.

DRUG FORMULARY

Every hospital should have a drug formulary. As per the policy of purchase of medicines, all medicines should be purchased only from the authorized dealers to avoid spurious drugs. The hospital authorities can ask the suppliers to submit the proof of their authority that they are genuine dealers of a particular company. The pharmacy or purchase department should buy the medicines mentioned in the drug formulary only.

Before preparing the drug formulary of the hospital, as it differs from hospital to hospital, the management should take the requirements of each consultant, medical departments, operation theater, etc.

In each generic medicine, the pharmacy can keep two or three brands of medicines. All the medicines can be listed in the book of drug formulary based on either diseasewise medicines or composition. But it should be easy to verify and find out the required medicine by the consultants.

Once the drug formulary is finalized by the management with the recommendations of the pharmacotherapeutic committee, all consultants have to follow the same while prescribing medicines to patients.

Any new drug is to be introduced or purchased on the requirement of consultant, tt can be done only after obtaining approval by the committee. The consultant sends his requirement for new drugs with the details of (i) the drug name, (ii) generic composition, (iii) strength of the drug, and (iv) usage of drug and the quantity required.

The pharmacist verifies the composition of new drug with available medicines and if it is not available or available with only one brand he will submit the requisition along with his remarks before the committee members and based on requirement, the committee will approve the new drugs. The management will send a circular to all consultants regarding the available of new drug in pharmacy and direct the pharmacist to keep stock of new drug in pharmacy. In case of any emergency, drugs can be procured by the pharmacy and the details should be submitted to the committee for ratification.

The drug formulary will be updated once in a year.

DRUG RECALL

Hundreds of pharmaceutical companies are manufacturing thousands of medicines in India. Most of the manufacturers are standard companies and are approved by the government authorities. But there are some spurious drugs in the market. The state or central government takes proper action on the companies producing these fake drugs, once it comes to the knowledge of the government.

The hospital management's duty and responsibility is to see that the branded and certified drugs alone should be purchased from the authorized dealers. Knowingly or unknowingly buying spurious and fake drugs leads to life threatening.

Inspite taking so many precautions sometimes some drugs may cause side effects which may badly affect the patients.

There are many reasons for side effects:

1. The patient may be allergic to a particular drug and if that drug is administered on him without knowing it she/he may develop some allergy and it can cure by giving antiallergic drugs.
2. The drug itself will have known side effects based on its composition. It may or may not produce any allergy to patients. This type of drugs may suit some patients and causes side effects to some patients. Doctors stop those drugs and prescribe alternate medicine even on the slight observation of reaction.
3. Sometimes patients are badly affected by the administration of wrong drugs, spurious drugs, contaminated drugs, and expired drugs. They may be very dangerous to the patients.

Irrespective of the reasons, if any drug adverse reaction is noticed/observed in the ward, the ward nurse should inform immediately to the pharmacy about the drug reaction.

She should inform the drugs name, batch number, expiry date to the Pharmacist. The pharmacist will recall the particular drug and inform all the wards to check and verify the stock of such drug and return it to the pharmacy. After proper verification the pharmacist will give directions to the ward for usage of the same.

If the ward nurse noticed any contamination in the bottle or IV fluids before giving to the patients, she should stop giving such drugs and inform to the pharmacist. Pharmacist will receive such drugs and return to the supplier on credit note. All drug adverse reaction should be reported and documented properly. It will be reviewed in the committee meetings.

CHAPTER 9

Dietetic Services

Though the canteen facility is a supporting service in a hospital, diet is as important as medicine for patient. Timely food to patients helps proper medication. Delay in the supply of food may lead to delay in medication.

The dieticians play an important role in dietetic service department. They work towards the object of providing tasty, hygienic and nutritionally balanced diet to patients as per their requirement and doctors' advice. They plan the diet for patient in coordination with the treating doctor.

The department serves the following types of food:

1. Normal food for patients.
2. Salt free food for blood pressure and renal failure patients.
3. Liquid or semisolid special diet for nasogastric and jejunostomy feeding patient.
4. Staff food either on concessional rate or normal rate.
5. Food for patient attendants.

CANTEEN ADMINISTRATION

1. The management can run the canteen for both patients and staff.
2. The management can run the canteen only for patients and give it on contract for staff food.
3. The management can outsource the canteen for both patients and staff. In case of 3rd option, management should monitor the patients' diet.

EFFECTIVE CANTEEN SERVICES

The following things must be done to enable efficient canteen services:

1. Appointment of qualified dieticians who have major role in patient diet.
2. Room service on time.

3. Right diet to right patient.
4. Late orders to be honored properly.
5. Maintainance of good quality and hygienic food.
6. Diet counseling to patient.
7. Supply of diet according to the patients' health condition.
8. Supply of food with required temperature.
9. Restriction of outside food except home food to prevent any food poisoning.
10. Install modern and automatic machines to minimize human handling.
11. Providing personal protective equipment like gloves, caps, aprons, etc.
12. Conducting periodical medical checkup for canteen staff who are handling food.
13. Smoking to be avoided in kitchen.
14. Use of quality of products for cleaning and washing utensils, floor area, etc.
15. Keeping the prepared food under cover and special care should be taken to control cockroaches, flies and mosquitoes.
16. Providing round the clock service at least for milk, coffee, bread, etc. for emergency patients and sick patients who require these products during nighttimes.
17. Keeping a raw material store nearest to the kitchen.
18. Providing adequate refrigerators or cold storage rooms for perishables.
19. Having a pest control schedule to prevent rats, cockroaches, flies, etc.
20. Provide good food trolleys, ovens, vessels, etc.
21. Hot cases and flasks to be cleaned properly or replaced periodically.
22. Correct billing, good system of inventory, bulk purchases on discount prizes, good cooling system for perishables, manpower planning, reduction of waste, etc. will help management to run kitchen effectively and profitably.

DUTIES AND RESPONSIBILITIES OF THE DIETICIAN

The dietician should deal with indoor as well outdoor patients.

The following are the procedures:

1. Getting the indoor patients' list morning from admitting clerk/reception.
2. Preparing standard diet sheets, in consultation with medical staff for special therapeutic diets like diabetic, low salt, low fat, gastric, reducing, etc.

3. Exercising supervision over preparation of such special diets.
4. Calculation of individual diet required for inpatients.
5. Compilation of weekly menus for patients.
6. Providing recipes for special dishes.
7. General training and detailed instructions to be given to cooks.
8. Visiting wards to interview and advise patients regarding their diets and to discuss dietetic problems with the ward sister.
9. Advising the supplying departments regarding the nutritive values and suitability of items to be procured, keeping in mind the need for economy.
10. Dietary surveys as desired by medical staff.
11. Diet counseling for inpatient and outpatients.
12. The prepared meals to be checked by the dieticians by actually tasting each dish before it is served to patients.
13. Dietician to maintain a register mentioning the daily report on the quality of the food served to the patients.
14. Planning patient diet as per the case history and discussions with the concerned consultants.
15. Diet slip to be prepared and given to the kitchen staff for disbursement of food as per their instructions.
16. The nutritional assessment and calculation of body mass index (BMI) to be done for both outpatient and inpatients.

CHAPTER 10

Hospital Infection Control

Hospital infection control (HIC) program is one of the major responsibilities of the top management in any hospital.

The aim of the hospital infection control program is to disseminate information, to conduct surveillance activities and investigations, prevention and control of nosocomial infections which affect approximately 2 million patients annually in acute care facilities in our country which costs several millions of rupees annually.

The quality of a hospital's infection control program is a reflection of the overall standard of care provided by that hospital. A good infection control program reduces nosocomial infections, length of patients stay in the hospital, and the costs associated with hospitalization.

Historically, infection control practices in one form or another have existed since great surgeons like Lister who recognized the significance of bacteria in producing postoperative wound infections. John Bell in 1801 remarked that hospital infection exists in every type of hospital.

In 1970s, the first infection control nurse was appointed in United Kingdom. This marked the beginning of an era and the recognition of infection controls as a speciality its own right.

COMPONENTS FOR EFFECTIVE INFECTION CONTROL PROGRAM

The following components should be included for effective infection control program.

1. Organized surveillance and control activities.
2. One infection control practitioner for every major hospital.

3. A trained hospital epidemiologist.
4. A system for reporting surgical wound infection rates and other infections back to the practicing surgeons and physicians.
5. Continuing education of medical staff.
6. Control of infectious disease outbreaks.
7. Protection of employee from infection.
8. Advice on new products, devices and procedures pertinent to infection control.
9. Instructions on all necessary control measures in the event of an outbreak or other infection control emergencies.

The healthcare-associated infections represent one of the most common complications of health care and are widely recognized as a major public health problem in both industrialized and developing countries. HIC programs are primarily dedicated to assisting the public health services—state and local health authorities' hospitals and other professional organizations in the prevention and control of nosocomial infections in the hospitals.

Since millions of patients are affected by nosocomial infections every year every hospital and healthcare provider should have an infection control system charged with monitoring, preventing and controlling the spread of infections in the healthcare environment.

Since the infection control requires the ability to detail infection when they occur the clinical microbiology laboratory should be linked with any comprehensive infectional control program.

PREDICTORS OF INFECTION

The important predictors of infection rate in hospitals are:

1. Intensity of surveillance.
2. Intensity of control measures.
3. One infection control practitioner/staff nurse for every 250 beds.
4. Presence of a trained infectious disease specialist on the staff.
5. Provision of SSI (surgical site infection) rates to surgeons.

GUIDELINES AND RECOMMENDATIONS FOR HIC PROGRAM

1. Handwashing and hospital environmental control.
2. Immunization.
3. Infectious disease control.
4. Intravascular device-related infections and its control.

5. Isolation precautions.
6. Long-term care facilities.
7. Guideline for infection control in healthcare personnel.
8. Surgical site infection control (SSI).
9. Urinary tract and respiratory tract infections control.
10. Bloodstream infections.
11. Hospital construction or modification.
12. Sterilization/disinfection.
13. Formulation, implementation and monitoring of antibiotic usage in the hospital by formulating an antibiotic policy.
14. The facility manager/maintenance supervisor should inform to the HIC team before taking up of the construction work in the premises, especially in the wards of the hospital for them to take necessary precaution to avoid infection.

HANDWASHING TECHNIQUES

Handwashing is one of the most important procedures for preventing nosocomial infections and washing is defined as a vigorous rubbing together of all surfaces of lathered hands followed by thorough rinsing under a stream of water.

Six steps are recommended in handwashing technique:

Step 1: Palm to palm.

Step 2: Palm of right hand over back of left hand palm of left hand over back of right hand.

Step 3: Palm to palm with fingers interfaced.

Step 4: Back of fingers to opposing palms with fingers interlocked.

Step 5: Rational rubbing of right thumb clasped in left palm and *vice versa.*

Step 6: Rational rubbing backwards and forwards with clasped fingers of right hand in left palm and *vice versa*.

Handwashing can be classified into two by the nature of the products used.

1. **Mechanical removal of microorganisms:**

   Handwashing with plain soaps or detergents (in bar, granule, leaflet or liquid form) suspends microorganisms and allows them to be rinsed off. This process is called mechanical removal of microorganisms.

2. Chemical removal of microorganism:

Handwashing with antimicrobial containing products kills or inhibits the growth of microorganisms. This process is called chemical removal of microorganisms.

HANDWASHING INDICATIONS

In the absence of true emergency, personnel should always wash their hands

- Before performing invasive procedures
- Before taking care of particularly susceptible patients such as those who are severely immuno compromised and newborn
- Before and after touching wounds whether surgical, traumatic or associated with an invasive device
- After situations during which microbial contamination of hands is likely to occur, especially those involving contract with mucous membranes blood or body fluids secretions or excretions
- After touching urine measuring devices or secretions collections apparatus
- After taking care of an infected patient
- Between contacts with different patients in high risk areas and all units.

Most routine activities involving direct/indirect patient contact other than that discussed above, e.g. taking blood pressure, handling a patient, medications, food or other objects, do not require handwashing.

HANDWASHING FACILITIES

- Handwashing facilities should be conveniently located throughtout the hospital.
- A sink should be located in or just outside every patient's room.
- Handwashing facilities should be located in or adjacent to rooms where diagnostic or invasive procedures that require hand washing are required.

STANDARD PRECAUTIONS

For procedures that are likely to generate splashes or sprays of body fluid a mask with eye protection or a face shield and a gown should be worn.

Recapping of needles should be discouraged.

HIC COMMITTEE

The Hospital Infection Control Committee consisting of a medial microbiologist, infectious diseases physician, medical and nursing superintendent, HIC nurse and hospital administrator, should meet monthly to discuss about HIC program. The meeting agenda should be well planned and circulated to committee members before the meeting.

FUNCTIONS OF THE COMMITTEE

The Committee performs three principle functions:
1. The first is to gather data or collect data.
2. The second function is to carry out surveillance.
3. The third function of the committee is to enforce good infection control practices.

The role of medical microbiologist is very much recognized in hospital infection control practices.

DUTIES AND RESPONSIBILITIES OF INFECTION CONTROL NURSE

- Daily rounds to critical care areas
- Educating and evaluating the staffs about infection control practices
- Handling/coordinating during outbreaks
- Monitoring, training, auditing and assurance of infection control activities like hand hygiene, biomedical waste management, adherence to universal precaution in the hospital among the healthcare workers
- Collection of data/analysis, root cause evaluation and corrective and preventive action for bundles on daily basis like,
  - Ventilator-Associated Pneumonia (VAP)
  - Catheter-Related Bloodstream Infection (CRBSI)
  - Catheter-Associated Urinary Tract Infection (CAUTI)
  - Surgical-Site Infection (SSI)

Reporting to the infection control committee.

- Periodical addressing all practical problems/issues related to infection control activities throughout the hospital
- Checking the adequacy of HIC related resources and coordinates with the respective HODs and top management for provision of resource to ensure smooth implementation of HIC practices
- Presenting the HAI status of the hospital in the HIC committee and also discussing the various issues related to resources/practices/implementation/documentation/results and Corrective And Preventive Action (CAPA)
- Reporting to HIC officer/doctor as per the frequency defined regarding the HIC status.

CHAPTER 11

Medical Gases

Different types of gases that are manufactured, packaged, and intended for administration to a patient in anaesthesia, therapy or diagnosis are called "medical gases".

TYPES OF MEDICAL GASES

Air, oxygen, nitrogen, nitrous oxide, carbon dioxide, and helium are the medical gases.

COLOR CODES FOR MEDICAL GASES

Color codes for medical gases as adopted by the bureau of standard of US are given below:

1. Air—yellow
2. Oxygen—green
3. Nitrogen—black
4. Nitrous oxide—blue
5. Carbon dioxide—gray
6. Helium—brown.

These medical gases can be supplied to wards, ICU, IMCU, OT etc through Central manifold system or though cylinders on trolley. Generally the multi- specialty hospital with more than 100 beds will have Central supply system. Sometimes it is viable to Centralize the supply of oxygen and other gases to OT and the rest of the hospital is supplied with medium size cylinders. In most of the hospitals oxygen and air (suction) are Centralized and others like nitrous oxide (N_2O) carbondioxide (CO_2), etc. are supplied by individual cylinders. This can be decided by the top Management depending upon the consumption of various gases. The industrial gases should not be used in hospitals.

USES AND PROPERTIES OF MEDICAL GASES

Gas	*Color code*	*Standard gauge pressure*	*Properties*	*Uses*
Oxygen	Green background White letter or White background With green letters	50–55 psi (345–380 kPa)	Tasteless/ colorless/ odorless Approx 21% of the atomosphere	Respiratory and inhalation therapy Used in conjunction with anesthesia machines, provide supplemental oxygen to the respiratory system, in dentistry in combination with nitrous oxide and as an emergency standby
Medical Air	Yellow background/black letters	50–55 psi (345–380 kPa)	Air consists of the approx gaseous volumes- 78.09% nitrogen, 20.95% oxygen, 0.93% argon, 0.03%, carbon dioxide, and minute traces of neon, helium, methane, krypon, hydrogen, xenon, and ozone	Respiratory therapy, drive ventilators, reduction of high oxygen concentrations, administering breathing treatments and as a mixing component for other respiratory gases
Medical/ surgical vacuum	White background/ black letters	15–30 in Hg (380–760 mmHg)	Result of pressure being less than atmospheric 0" Hg gauge = atmospheric pressure (i.e. 0 vacuum) while 30" Hg gauge = perfect vacuum	Assists in draining fluids and tissue from patients. The medical vacuum infrastructure is designed to remain dry

Contd...

Contd...

Gas	*Colour Code*	*Standard gauge pressure*	*Properties*	*Uses*
Nitrogen	Black background/ white letters	160–185 psi (1100–1275 kPa)	Colorless/ odorless approx 78% of the atmosphere	Power pneumatic tools, provide pneumatic pressure in medical equipment; to present combustion and other chemical reactions; and a component of many gas mixtures
Nitrous oxide (also called laughing gas)	Blue background/ white letters	50–55 psi (345–380 kPa)	Colorless with sweetish taste and odor, supports combustion	Analgesic agent (diverse group of drugs used to relieve plain), used in anesthesia, used as an anesthetic agent in surgery, mixed with oxygen to help patients relax during dental procedures; and in cryosurgery (the use of extreme cold to destroy tissues)
Carbon dioxide	Gray background/black letters or gray background/white letters	160–185 psi (1100–1275 kPa)	Colorless/ odorless/ Tasteless, appox 0.03% of the atmosphere, does not support combustion (other than when combined with magnesium)	Stimulates respiration, used in insufflations (expands a body cavity by blowing carbon dioxide in to it)

Contd...

Contd...

Gas	*Colour Code*	*Standard gauge pressure*	*Properties*	*Uses*
WAGD (Waste Anesthetic Gas Disposal)	Violet background/ white Letters	Can vary with the system type used	Result of pressure being less than atmospheric. "0" in Hg gauze = atmospheric pressure (i.e. 0 vacuum) while 30 in Hg gauge = perfect vacuum	Removal of anesthesia Gases expelled from a patient.
Instrument air	Red back ground/ white letters	160–185 psig (1100–1275 kPa)	Air consists of the approx gaseous volumes – 78.09% nitrogen, 20.95% oxygen, 0.93% argon. 0.03% carbon dioxide, and minute traces of neon, helium, methane, krypton, hydrogen, xenon, and ozone	Power pneumatic tools.
Helium	Brown			Used in breathing mixtures for patients with impaired lung functions and in MRI scan

PROCEDURES FOR PURCHASE OF MEDICAL GASES

1. The hospital should purchase medical gases from an agency with license to do business with medical gases.
2. Normally the agency will supply in its own cylinders or rented basis. The empty ones will be given back and the filled cylinders are received from the agency.
3. If a hospital owns these cylinders, the agency will fill the cylinders and bring them back to the hospital.
4. If a hospital owns the cylinders, they should be sent for inspection periodically as specified by the agency. The inspection certificate should be preserved.
5. At the time of purchasing a new cylinder the explosive certificates/ fitness certificate should be obtained from the regulatory authorities.
6. If a hospital goes for central systems the following points should be considered:
   a. To decide whether hospital requires only wall outlets or flexible pendants also in the OT.
   b. To go for a suitable wall terminal unit that will not allow leakage and it is to operate by nurses and other paramedical staff.
   c. The central system to have zonal isolation valves. It allows cutting of service of one area without affecting other area of supply. It helps during maintenance and also cuts wastage if one area is not used for long time.
   d. To have an alarm system to indicate the pressure in pipelines. It also indicates that supply has changed from normal to standby.
   e. The Central gas manifold unit to consist of (i) control panel, (ii) right and left bank of cylinders for oxygen and N_2O (iii) stand by management for emergency purpose.
7. Individual oxygen cylinder should not be used without properly fitting with oxygen therapy accessories, oxygen regulators, flow meter and humidifier.
8. If a hospital uses individual cylinders, proper checking is required as mentioned below:
   a. All the medical gas cylinders should be checked by the pressure of gas in it. Fix the pressure gauge in the cylinder and check the pressure.
   b. The standard pressure for all medical gases was already given in this chapter.
   c. Nitrous oxide cylinder must be checked by weight.

DUTIES AND RESPONSIBILITY OF MANIFOLD OPERATOR

1. He should ensure that all the cylinders in the manifold room are intact.
2. He should open the number of cylinders to ensure the correct pressure in the pipe line.
3. He should use cylinders from one side of the manifold cylinder bank (right side or left side).
4. The empty cylinders of one side of manifold should be sent for refilling.
5. He should check all cylinders for leakage by using soap water mixture.
6. He should maintain stock of required tools in the manifold rooms.
7. He should take a round of the hospital to see all the outlets are properly functioning.
8. He should rectify or arrange to repair any defects in the pipeline, outlets or in the manifold room.
9. He should take care of supply of O_2 and other gases in other areas where there is no central pipeline.
10. Replacement of empty cylinders with loaded cylinders in the wards should be done.
11. All the major problems should be brought to the notice of the administrators immediately.

SAFETY MEASURES TO BE TAKEN

FIRE AND EXPLOSION

All flammable gases and even nonflammable gases should be stored in the absence of a source of ignition. Special attention should be paid to smoking, electrical spares and even to static electricity.

STORAGE

- Cylinders should be stored inside, under cover, not exposed to extreme cold and heat
- Cylinders should be kept dry, clean and ventilated at top and bottom
- Cylinders should not be stored near combustible stores
- Full and empty cylinders should be kept separate
- Cylinders should not be allowed to become rust and dirty and should never be repainted, nor their markings observed
- No smoking, warning sign boards must be provided
- There should be good access to the store for delivery vehicle.

HANDLING

- Cylinders should be handled gently and should not be knocked violently
- They should be moved with the appropriate trolley
- When moved, cylinder valve must be closed.

LEAKS

- Leak is usually evident because of its hissing noise
- The location of the leak can be found by bruising suspected area with soap water and noting the formation of bubbles

IN USE

- Cylinders should be firmly secured to a suitable support or contained in a stand or trolley and in vertical position
- Smoking and naked light should never be allowed near cylinder.

AFTER USE

Cylinder valve should be closed firmly with just sufficient force after use.

PRECAUTIONS FOR USE

- The valves should be opened momentarily and closed to blow away any of foreign matter, making sure that the handless face is not in front.
- Ensure that the connecting face of the regulator is clean.
- Use only a reasonable amount of effort to tighten the connecting while attaching regulator.
- Cylinders should always be used in conjunction with pressure regulator.
- Cylinders valves and associated equipment must never be lubricated and should be kept entirely free from oil and grease.

The important key indicator for the department is to ensure continuous supply of medical gases to wards, OT, etc. without any interruption and to ensure correct pressure in pipeline.

CHAPTER 12

Consent

Consent is defined as:

"Two or more persons are said to consent when they agree upon the same thing in the same sense" (Sec 13, The Indian Contract Act). For the purpose of clinical examination, diagnosis and treatment, any person who is conscious, mentally sound and is above 18 years of age can give consent. Consent is not legally valid when given under fear, fraud or misrepresentation of facts.

TYPES OF CONSENT

i. Implied consent.
ii. Express consent, which may be verbal consent or written consent.
iii. Informed consent.

IMPLIED CONSENT

This is most common type of consent in both general practice and hospital practice. The fact that a patient comes to a doctor for an ailment implies that he is agreeable to medical examination in general sense. In clinical practice, implied consent can be used for general examination and systemic examination, including inspection, palpation, percussion and auscultation.

EXPRESSED CONSENT

This type of consent is used when a patient specifically grants permission to a physician to undertake diagnosis and treatment of a specific problem. Expressed consent may be given either verbally or in writing. Expressed consent must conform to the doctrine of informed consent to be legally acceptable. Once a patient has forbidden any action, the question of implied consent does not arise.

Expressed written consent should be obtained for the following:

i. All invasive and major diagnostic procedures
ii. General anesthesia
iii. Surgical operations
iv. Medicolegal examinations for determining age, potency, virginity, etc. where the person being examined is not in police custody.

DOCTRINE OF INFORMED CONSENT

The doctrine of informed consent aims at giving sufficient information to a patient to enable him to make a knowledgeable and informed decision about the use of a drug, device or procedure in the course of treatment. The duty to warn a patient of any likely harm in the course of treatment has also been included in the doctrine. In order to conform to the doctrine of informed consent, the following conditions should be fulfilled:

i. Disclosure of information
ii. Free and voluntary decision-making by the patient
iii. The legal competency of the patient to decide.

The treating physician must ensure that the patient is explained the following in a language he/she understands:

i. Provisional diagnosis
ii. Nature of procedure/treatment
iii. Risks involved
iv. Prospect of success
v. Likely outcome in case the procedure is not performed
vi. Alternative methods of treatment.

SITUATIONS WHERE CONSENT IS NOT REQUIRED

Consent is not required to be obtained in the following situations:

i. Medical emergencies: consent to emergency treatment is implied.
ii. Treatment of notifiable diseases: in the interest of public health.
iii. Medical examination under Sec 53, Cr PC.
iv. Psychiatric examination/treatment by court order.

Under Section 53 (1) of Cr PC, a person can be examined at request of the police by use of force. Section 53 (2) lays down that whenever a female is to be examined, it shall be done only by or under the supervision of a female doctor.

As far as possible, consent must be obtained from the patient, when he/she is competent to give it. Consent to treatment or a procedure or an operation is limited to the parameters that were expressed before the commencement of medical intervention. However, in certain circumstances, extension of the scope of consent would be legally permissible. This principle of extension applies in cases of consent to treat an emergency. Consent should be obtained when procedure has finally been decided and planned and not while the investigation is still contemplated. Consent should be obtained in the presence of a witness before preoperative medication is administered and the same is documented in writing. Only in situations where the patient is minor, unconscious or mentally unsound, consent should come from legal guardian/Near of Kith and Kin (NOK), who are present. In case of an unconscious patient, consent to emergency treatment is Implied.

Legally, it is essential to take consent for the following reasons:

i. It provides a practitioner legal protection in case of an action for negligence. The practitioner can cite proof of consent as evidence of disclosure, thereby protecting him from an action based on failure to disclose material facts.

ii. Secondly, protection has been provided to practitioners who have obtained informed consent in accordance with the provisions of Sec 88, I.P.C.

iii. Thirdly, it may be pertinent to note that exercise of reasonable skill and care is not sustainable in law as a defense against assault and battery.

CHAPTER 13

Operation Theaters

Operation theaters (OTs) are one of the important high risk areas in the hospital. Multispecialty hospitals are not complete without operation theatres. There should be a minimum of two operation theatres in any hospital. The multispecialty hospitals will have separate operation theatres for the following specialties:

a. Cardiothoracic surgery
b. Ophthalmology
c. Renal transplantation
d. Liver transplantation
e. Obstetric and gynecological procedures
f. Neurosurgeries
g. General surgical procedures
h. Infected cases
i. Minor procedures.

POINTS FOR EFFECTIVE FUNCTIONING OF OTs

The operation theaters should be fully equipped with good OT light, OT table, ventilators, etc. They should also have facilities like central air-conditioning, central medical gas system, etc.

The minor OT should be provided near OPD/emergency for routine small procedures.

During an emergency, this OT can be used as a labor room also. Otherwise the labor theater is always a dedicated well equipped room.

The postoperative wards should be located near the OT complex.

The surgical procedures will be carried out in the theaters as mentioned above.

The operation theater complex should be designed in such a way that there should be a minimum of two barriers of entry.

The first barrier of OT should not be crossed without changing the shoes and slippers.

The second barrier should not be crossed without changing of dress.

This should be strictly followed by one and all including surgeons.

The OT area should be kept sterilized.

Proper care should be taken while constructing operation theaters especially regarding walls and floor of the theaters.

The walls of the major theatre should be such that cleaning of walls is easy. The walls should be painted with plastic paint or tiles or marble or granite and it should be put up to total height of all four walls. But there should not be any gaps between the tiles or it should be minimum to avoid formation of dust particles between the tiles.

Similarly, the flooring should be antistatic to avoid any mishap in OT. The flooring can be done by using SL epoxy static dissipative material or marble or granite materials.

Some of the hospitals are making sophisticated modular state-of-art operation theaters with stainless steel walls, roofs, pendents and doors. The stainless steel walls and roofs are joint free and it is easy to clean and wash with disinfectants.

OT should be fumigated every week or fortnight and after every septic surgery.

Cultures should be taken after fumigation and the reports should be kept. Samples for culture should be collected from the four corners of OT, Boyl's machine, OT table, walls (four feet above the ground level) and from the air.

CRITERIA FOR A GOOD OT AIR CONDITIONING

The following points are to be considered for a good OT air-conditioning

1. OT size: The recommended size of the OT is 22 × 18 × 10 (L × B × H). But it can be of any size which can accommodate OT equipments with a free space to move by the surgeons and other OT staff.
2. Equipment load: The total number of equipment that are available in OT with their power consumption should be considered.
3. Ambient temperature and humidity: Before designing A/C plant for OT the ambient temperature at peak condition of 41–42°C and the humidity at 55°F (15) should be considered.

4. Air changes per hour: The fresh air entry air changes per hour should be calculated.
5. Air velocity: Vertical down flow diffusers and unidirectional flow with downwards to the ground should be considered. The air flow on the diffusers should be measured.
6. Positive pressure: It should be measured with a monometer and found the number of Pascal maintained.
7. Air handling units: The air should be supplied through the HEPA filters in the ceiling. The filtration area, air volume, return air grills, the quality of air, etc. should be considered.
8. The laminar air flow is required for major OT to avoid infections.
9. Dual operation theaters should be planned for any transplant surgeries like renal transplantation, liver transplantation and heart transplantation.

COMMON EQUIPMENTS AVAILABLE IN OT

1. Shadow less OT light
2. OT table
3. Boyl's machine
4. Ventilator
5. Defibrillator
6. Monitor (Multiparameter)
7. Suction machine
8. Surgical diathermy machine
9. C-Arm
10. ECG machine
11. Syringe pump
12. Nebulizer
13. BP
14. Ambu bag
15. Laryngoscope
16. Thermometer
17. Stethoscope
18. Fumigator
19. Pendents
20. Needle destroyer
21. Microscope
22. Surgical instruments
23. Heart lung machine (for CTOT).

CHECKLIST BEFORE STARTING ANY PROCEDURE

1. Status of OT sterilization
2. Status of linen with sterilization indicator
3. Status of surgical instruments
4. Status of medical gases
5. Physical checking of suction trolley
6. Physical checking of various equipments
7. Physical checking of anesthesia machine
8. Physical checking of all electrical outlets
9. Physical checking of A/C and ventilation

10. Physical checking of all listed drugs and disposables
11. Physical checking of scrub station
12. Availability of dresses and slippers
13. Checking correct name of the patient
14. Checking the type of surgery and site of surgery
15. Checking preanesthesia check-up report
16. Checking the consent forms.

DUTIES AND RESPONSIBILITIES OF OT IN-CHARGE

1. OT in-charge should keep all necessary drugs and disposables in the OT.
2. He/she should also maintain an inventory of drugs, instruments and other equipments in OT.
3. He/she should be responsible for proper care and maintenance of OT equipments and to ensure that they are always in working order.
4. He/she should contact the suppliers for periodical maintenance/service of OT equipments.
5. He/she should maintain a record for loss/breakage/damage of any equipment or OT items and it should be reported to the administration.
6. He/she should practice and monitor continuously the sterilization procedures in OT.
7. Adverse bacteriological results should be brought to the notice of the surgeon/microbiologist immediately.
8. He/she should also take remedial action for adverse bacteriological results.
9. He/she should not permit unauthorized staff in the OT.
10. He/she should maintain the operation list, for each day in advance without any clash between two surgeons.
11. She should maintain discipline among the staff working in OT.
12. She should be responsible for allotment of duties to OT staff.
13. She should also be responsible for arranging staff, round the clock to attend on emergency surgeries.
14. She should assist surgeons/anaesthetists at operations as required by them.
15. She should be responsible for preparation of OT bill for OT charges, items used in OT, instrument charges, etc. and she should send the same to the billing section.
16. She should be also responsible to run the theater economically and avoid wastage.

In addition to the above duties and responsibilities the OT in-charge should maintain the dignity and decorum of the profession and should be at all times be cheerful, kind, courteous and sympathetic towards patients and to their anxious relatives. The qualities along with professional skills will win the respect and cooperation of patients.

DUTIES AND RESPONSIBILITIES OF OT TECHNICIAN/NURSE

1. General cleanliness of the theater and its sterilization.
2. Preparation of sets and sterilizing them before the end of the day.
3. Preparing for the next day surgery before leaving the hospital.
4. Care of equipments and cleaning of instruments.
5. Maintenance of operation register.
6. Return of medical records to the ward along with the patient after surgery.
7. Getting operative notes completed by the surgeons.
8. To attend on emergency duties.
9. Assisting OT in-charge with other administrative work, like maintaining inventories, etc.
10. Following the instruction given by OT in-charge.

CHAPTER 14

Blood Bank

DEFINITION OF BLOOD BANK

A place where blood is collected from the voluntary donors, labeled with blood group, and into components, stored and prepared for transfusion to patients. A blood bank or blood transfusion service may be a autonomous facility or part of a larger laboratory in a hospital.

OBJECTIVE OF THE DEPARTMENT OF BLOOD TRANSFUSION MEDICINE

To provide appropriate, high quality, safe blood/blood components, to the patients by collecting blood from the voluntary blood donors.

FUNCTIONS

- To supply adequate and appropriate blood and blood products in a timely manner
- To provide specialist support and advise in matters relating to transfusion medicine
- To strive for excellence in all aspects in transfusion medicine
- To provide a convenient, caring and safe environment for donors, staff and public
- To minimize any adverse environmental impact resulting in blood transfusion service operation
- To actively recruit and retain voluntary donors to donate blood and blood components
- To collect blood from selected donors, screen it for known transfusion Infectious diseases and correctly determine its blood group

- To prepare and provide blood and blood components essential for use in modern medical treatment
- To store and distribute blood and blood products to patients throughout in a timely and efficient manner on a 24 hours availability basis
- To provide limited therapeutic services
- To facilitate applied development and clinical research
- To educate nursing, scientific and medical fraternities, and the general public, about blood transfusion and related technology
- To provide a specialist library, technical reference service and training in transfusion science and medicine.

DUTIES AND RESPONSIBILITIES OF BLOOD BANK MEDICAL OFFICER

- Checking at the beginning of the day whether all the consumables, chemicals, reagents and kits available and in sufficient quantity
- Keeping the department clean
- Check whether the test requisition form is filled in all fields and contains all the necessary details, namely name, age, sex, ID number, tests requested, date and time of collection the sample and signature of the nursing staff/ collection center technician who collected the sample
- Using closed containers for transporting the samples from the wards
- Generating a separate lab ID number for IP and outside samples received for testing
- Rejecting samples even with any one of the following:
  - Samples, which are hemolyzed/decomposed
  - Insufficient sample
  - Samples without an ID number/decomposed.
- Do not centrifuge the samples in uncapped vacutainer tubes
- Bringing the reagent, chemicals, and kits to room temperature before use
- Checking the expiry date of the reagents and kits before use as they should not be used beyond expire date. In case of expiry or non-availability of test kits, tests have to be sent to a accredited laboratory as temporary measure
- Processing all requests for blood bank tests on the same day within 2 hours of collection. For tests, which are not done immediately should be separated the serum and allot them in storage vials with a label indicating the ID number and the tests to be done until the time of testing

- Running positive and negative control whenever a new batch/lot of reagent used
- The final report shall be handed over to the technician of the blood bank department who verifies it for any transcription errors such as spelling mistakes, misplaced decimal points
- Retaining all processed samples for seven days before discarding
- Following are the personnel protection and safety measures while performing tests:
  - Segregating and disposing all the biohazardous and nonbiohazardous materials and the processed samples as per 'treatment of biomedical waste'
  - Storing the reagents and kits in use in the refrigerator within the department at the temperature as specified by the manufacturer in the product insert
  - Recording the details of equipment maintenance breakdown and any preventive maintenance carried out in the machine history record and calibration record.
- Calibrating all the measuring and testing equipment used in the department as per departmental calibration plan and recording the details in the equipment calibration record
- Taking a stock of all the reagents and kits at the end of every month form the details in the stock register—blood banks
- Placing an indent for the consumables required by filling the necessary details in the purchase requisition form (PRF) for approval by the head of the department and sending the same to the purchase department.

Stamping an inspection seal on the delivery challan when the items are received at the department. The receiver of the item is to check for any damage, date of expiry, seal. If the item is accepted a signature is made on the delivery challan and a copy of the same is sent to the materials/ central purchase department and the other copy is placed in the delivery challan file.

Inspecting the stock received for acceptance and if found not suitable for use, inform the supplier through the central purchase department and record the details in the purchase register.

Providing the necessary training to all the employees working in the department according to the training requirements.

BLOOD AND BLOOD DONATION

1. WHAT IS BLOOD?

Blood is made of straw-colored fluid called plasma, in which many tiny cells are suspended. These are mostly red blood cells, with some white cells and smaller cells called platelets. Total blood volume: 60–80 mL/kg. The rest is fluid.

2. WHAT IS THE ROLE OF RED BLOOD CELLS?

The red blood cells are given their color by a pigment called hemoglobin. This is a complex protein, containing iron, which is found in no other cells. The red blood cells carry oxygen from air in the lungs to all the cells of the body. The waste product called carbon dioxide is picked up by cells and plasma and brought back from the tissues to the lungs where it s once more exchanged for oxygen.

3. WHAT IS THE ROLE OF WHITE BLOOD CELLS?

The white blood cells protect the body against infection. Some white cells fight bacteria by surrounding and then destroying them, while others build up the body's immunity to diseases. They also act as scavenger cells in removing injured tissue or small particles of foreign materials.

4. WHAT IS THE FUNCTION OF PLATELETS?

Platelets are necessary for the formation of blood clots, thus helping to reduce blood loss from the wounds.

5. WHAT IS THE FUNCTION OF PLASMA?

Plasma contains water, minerals and other substances absorbed from food for supply to all the cells in the body. It carries hormones and transports waste products to the kidneys for excretion. Plasma also contains many proteins, including blood clotting factors and immunoglobulins (anti bodies). Many of these proteins can now be separated from blood: some are used to treat patients with deficiencies of these substances. There are more than 13 important blood clotting factors.

6. WHO CAN DONATE BLOOD?

A healthy person between the ages of 18 and 65 years can donate blood. Under 18s need parental consent, on the form provided by the blood bank.

Donors should have a weight of minimum of 45 kg and must NOT be in a risk category for AIDS, and other diseases transmissible by blood. A first time donor must be under the age of 65 years.

7. HOW MUCH BLOOD IS TAKEN FROM THE DONOR?

One unit of blood is approximately 450 ml/350 ml. or about 9% of an adult's blood volume.

8. HOW MUCH BLOOD DOES THE BODY HAS?

The average adult has about 5 liters of blood flowing through the body (Range).

9. HOW LONG DOES IT TAKE TO CARRY THE BLOOD?

The donation only takes about 45 minutes but you need to allow approximately once in every three months (or approximately every 2200 hours) should be allowed to give someone else another chance of life.

10. HOW LONG DOES IT TAKE THE BODY TO REPLACE THE BLOOD?

It takes the body 24–28 hours to replace the plasma portion which is about 80% water and 3–5 weeks to replace the red cells. Donors are encouraged to drink plenty of nonalcoholic fluid before and after donation and assist this process.

11. HOW OFTEN CAN BLOOD BE DONATED?

Donors can donate/give blood every 12 weeks depending on the health of the person.

12. SHOULD ONE EAT BEFORE GIVING BLOOD?

Yes, a substantial meal can be taken between one to four hours before donating in order to avoid any tendency to faint. Also plenty of water before and after donation can be consumed.

13. WHY SHOULD A DONOR REST AFTER GIVING BLOOD?

The rest period allows the body to adjust to the loss of blood in the system and for the blood transfusion service to ensure the bleeding has stopped before the donor leaves the donation area.

14. WHY IS A SMALL SAMPLE OF BLOOD TAKEN BEFORE DONATING?

A sample of blood is taken from the donor's finger to check the hemogolobin content. This test indicates whether the donor has a enough level hemoglobin to donate.

15. WHY HE SHOULD FILL UP A QUESTIONNAIRE ON AIDS?

The AIDS questionnaire is the first part of the screening procedure to reduce the possibility of taking blood from someone infected with HIV (AIDS) virus.

16. WHAT TESTS ARE DONE ON THE BLOOD AFTER IT HAS BEEN DONATED?

Every donation is checked in the virus serology laboratory for hepatitis B and hepatitis C, ALT, HTLV1, syphilis and the AIDS virus antibody. While these tests are in progress, the grouping laboratory identifies the ABO and rhesus groupings of that donation.

17. WHAT ARE BLOOD GROUPS?

Blood groups are inherited from both parents just like height, eye color, etc. The group is divided into 2 parts, the ABO part (with A,B,O or AB) and the rhesus part. The rhesus part gives us the 'positive or negative'.

18. WHAT ARE THE MOST COMMON AND LEAST COMMON BLOOD GROUPS?

The most common blood group is O positive, the least common group is AB negative.

19. WHO CAN RECEIVE WHICH GROUP?

Patients who are to receive blood have a sample of their blood cross matched with a sample of the donor's blood to ensure compatibility. Normally, patients will receive blood of the same ABO and Rh group although in an emergency, group O negative blood may be given to a patient of another group. If a patient is given blood which is incompatible, it may lead to his death.

20. DO DONORS GET PAID MONEY TO GIVE BLOOD?

No. Giving blood is a voluntary act by people who wish to help others.

21. DO PATIENTS HAVE TO PAY FOR BLOOD?

Patients are not charged for the blood they receive. However, they may be charged by the hospital for testing carried out by the hospital on their behalf.

PRECAUTIONS TO BE TAKEN FOR BLOOD TRANSFUSION AMONG BLOOD RELATIVES

First degree relative of the patient is not encouraged for blood donation. They can give as voluntary donors for other patients, if still they want to transfuse their blood for their relations, leukocyte deplection and gamma irradiation to be done on that particular blood component.

Leukocyte depletion significantly reduce the risk of transmission of cytomegalovirus (CMV).

Technically speaking geriatic patients, pediatric patients, immunocompromised patients, 100% gamma irradiation and leukodeplection should be done. If not patient may develop GVHD (graft versus host disease).

CHAPTER 15

Medical Record Department

Medical record department (MRD) is one of the most important department in a multispecialty hospital. The entire medical records and case-sheet of patients will be stored and maintained in MRD. The staff of MRD are busy in interacting with doctors and ward nurses to provide necessary information about the patient. The MRD should have a separate place for doctors to come and verify or to discuss the patients case history. One of the important function of MRD staff is the retrieval of patients data from the files as per the requirement of doctors. They not only maintain the data but they also analyze the data and prepare monthly statements as per the policy of the administration.

The building of patients case papers starts at the time of admission in main reception. It starts with the collection of personal details of a patient by the receptionist.

The case-sheet of a patient comprises of many forms starting from patient personal details, case-history, nurses notes, doctor's note, charge-sheet, etc.

All consent forms will also be filed in case-sheet. The staff nurse in charge of the ward should file all the documents related to that particular patient during the treatment period.

At the time of discharge case-sheet of a particular patient who is getting discharge should be sent to reception/billing section as per the system of the hospital for preparation of final bill.

The billing staff will make all charges mentioned in the case-sheet in final bill and send back the case-sheet to the ward.

The ward in-charge should file the discharge summary of a patient signed by the treating doctor and resident medical officer and check all the documents. The case-sheetshould be sent to medical record department after making necessary entries in the handing over register.

The staff in MRD should receive all case-sheets of patients discharged on the same day or previous next day.
The ward in-charge should not keep the case-sheet of a patient, who has already discharged, for not more than 24 hours in the ward.
The MRD should maintain all the case-sheets of hospital patients in order to enable the staff to take the case-sheet immediately without any delay. The case-sheet of medicolegal cases should be maintained separately. As per the policy of the hospital the case-sheet of death cases also should be maintained separately.
The old records of a patient should be issued to the ward, either for Doctors verification or for readmission, only through the procedure laid down by the management.

SOME OF THE IMPORTANT FORMS WHICH ARE TO BE FILLED IN PATIENT CASE-SHEET BEFORE SENDING IT TO THE MRD

1. Patient information sheet/initial assessment chart
2. Clinical chart
3. Nurses note
4. Doctors note
5. Intake and outtake chart
6. Drug chart
7. Neuro chart
8. Ventilator chart
9. Critical care chart
10. Investigation chart
11. Progress sheet
12. Dialysis charges chart
13. Discharge summary/death summary.

For Surgical Cases

14. Preoperative check list
15. Preanesthetist assessment
16. Anesthetic record
17. Operation record
18. Recovery room chart
19. Consent forms.

In addition to the above forms any other forms introduced by the hospital administration should be filled in the case-sheet.

DUTIES AND RESPONSIBILITIES OF MEDICAL RECORD OFFICER

1. The medical record officer should be responsible to the CMD/MS/hospital administrators.
2. Should check that the MRD has received files of all the discharged patients within 24 hours from the time of discharge.
3. He/she shall maintain a MRD record register, where he/she will be entering the files received in order of MRD or IP numbers.
4. If he/she has not received a file of a discharged patient, it will be his/her duty to find out the reason and search for missing file.
5. If not traced, the matter should be brought to the knowledge of CMD/MS/administrators.
6. If it is lost, an entry should be made in the MRD register giving actual reasons.
7. Should make sure that all records and forms are filled properly before keeping file in a rack.
8. If the records are not filled in the case-sheet, it is his/her duty to get the deficiency cleared by the concerned person.
9. Should complete or get completed various columns of case-sheet from admission to discharge of the patient.
10. Should be aware of the WHO International Classification of Diseases (ICD) and should code the disease of discharged patients.
11. Should be responsible for completing "birth and death register" and send information to municipal authorities.
12. Should receive all MLC case-sheets and injury registers from respective departments.
13. Should pay special attention to see that all MLC records are complete and kept separate under lock and key or in a secured place.
14. Should be responsible for providing all assistance to police officers, Insurance investigations and court pensions in collecting information of the patient through the case-sheet.
15. Should provide the required information to the above mentioned persons after obtaining approval from the CMO/MS/administrators.
16. He/she will be responsible to attend court and produce required record. Received on behalf of the hospital management.
17. Should prepare periodical reports like:
    a. Occupancy details
    b. Number of admissions and discharges

c. International classification of disease wise patients admitted report
d. List of number of deficiencies found in case-sheet and rectification report
e. Number of discharges unitwise, areawise, wardwise, etc.
f. Average length of stay of patients
g. Number of MLC patients discharged
h. Details of births and deaths
i. Details of patients admitted with notifiable diseases.

18. Should make sure that the department works efficiently and smoothly
19. Should perform any other duties/responsibilities assigned by the management.

For the purpose of the calculating the statistical ratio of utilization of hospital services different formulae's are given below. It is one of the duty of medical record officer (MRO) to calculate various ratios and submit to the management periodically. This data will help the management to review the performance of the departments and the quality of services given to the patients.

BED OCCUPANCY RATE

1. Ratio of actual patient days to the maximum possible patient days during a given period.
2. Ratio of the average daily census to the bed complement

$$\text{BOR} = \frac{\text{Average daily census}}{\text{Bed complement}} \times 100$$

BED TURNOVER RATE (BTR)

Bed turnover rate gives the number of discharges per hospital bed over a given period, i.e. how many times a bed was "turned over" during the period, say a year. It is directly related to the average length of stay (ALS) and bed turnover interval (BTI)

$$\frac{\text{Total number of patients discharged (including deaths)}}{\text{Bed complement}}$$

BED TURNOVER INTERVAL (BTI)

It denotes the average time in days elapsing between the discharge of one patient and the admission of the next on that bed.

$$\text{BTI} = \frac{\text{Potential no. of hospitalization days} - \text{Actual number of hospitalization days}}{\text{Number of discharges (including deaths)}}$$

e.g. $$\frac{1{,}09{,}500 - 98{,}200}{5{,}680} = 1.9$$

For 300 beds $300 \times 365 = 10{,}9500$

Actual $269 \times 365 = 98{,}200$

which means that each bed remained vacant during the year for an average of 1.9 days between on discharge and the next admission on that bed.

AVERAGE LENGTH OF STAY

Average length of stay (ALS) is the average period in hospital (in days) per patient admitted, i.e. the average number of days of service rendered to each inpatient.

$$\text{ALS} = \frac{\text{Number of inpatient days care (excluding Healthy newborn) during the year}}{\text{Total number of discharges and deaths}}$$

For 300 beds, 50% occupancy

$$\text{ALS} = \frac{150 \times 365}{\text{No. of discharges}} = \frac{54750}{\text{No. of discharges and deaths}}$$

HOSPITAL ADMISSION RATE

Hospital admission rate denotes the number of hospital admissions per 1000 population per year

$$\text{Hospital admission rate} = \frac{\text{Total admission during the year}}{\text{Mid year population}} \times 1000$$

PER CAPITA HOSPITALIZATION RATE

Per capita hospitalization rate is the per capita days of hospital care given for a particular gerographical area, during a particular period. It express the volume of hospitalization in terms of number of hospitalization days per person per year.

$$\frac{\text{Total number of days of inpatient care}}{\text{Mid year population}}$$

DAILY AVERAGE OUTPATIENT ATTENDANCE

$$\frac{\text{Total number of outpatient attendance during the period}}{\text{Number of OPD working days during the period}}$$

AVERAGE OUTPATIENT ATTENDANCE PER PATIENT

$$\frac{\text{Total number of outpatient attendances}}{\text{Total number of new cases}}$$

GROSS DEATH RATE

$$= \frac{\text{No. of all deaths in a period}}{\text{No. of discharges including deaths in the period}} \times 100$$

NET DEATH RATE

$$= \frac{\text{No. of deaths occurring 48 hr or later}}{\text{No. of deaths and discharges}} \times 100$$

POSTOPERATIVE DEATH RATE

$$= \frac{\text{No. of postoperative deaths in a period}}{\text{No. of patients operated during the period}} \times 100$$

MATERNAL DEATH RATE

These are the deaths of mother attributable to pregnancy, childbirth or its complication including death resulting from abortions

$$= \frac{\text{No. of deaths of obstetrical patients}}{\text{No. of discharges of obstetric patients}} \times 100$$

INFANT DEATH RATE (VIABLE INFANTS ABOUT 28 WEEKS)

$$= \frac{\text{No. of deaths of infants born in hospital}}{\text{No. of viable newborn infants (including deaths)}} \times 100$$

NEONATAL DEATH RATE

$$= \frac{\text{No. of infant deaths within 28 days or birth}}{\text{No. of viable newborn infants discharged}} \times 100$$

AUTOPSY RATE

This relates to autopsies carried out on patients who died in hospital. It excludes stillbirths, cases dead on arrival/brought dead, and medicolegal cases.

$$= \frac{\text{No. of autopsies}}{\text{No. of deaths in hospital}} \times 100$$

CONSULTATION RATE

$$= \frac{\text{No. of patients coming for consultations after discharge}}{\text{No. of patients discharged}} \times 100$$

CESAREAN SECTION RATE

$$= \frac{\text{No. of cesarean section performed}}{\text{No. of births}} \times 100$$

CHAPTER 16

Biomedical Engineering Department

Equipment used to evaluate the parameters of human body functions and machines used electrical signal to get the image of internal organs are called as diagnostic biomedical equipment. These equipments do not change or alter any parameter of the physiological function of the body, but give the physician enough data to assess the present condition of a patient.

SOME OF THE EQUIPMENTS

Some of the equipments are as follows:

AMBU BAG

It is a self refilling bag with 1.0–1.5 L capacity of air used for artificial respiration.

BOYLE'S ANESTHESIA APPARATUS

It is a continuous flow gas-oxygen anesthetic machine, used to make the patient loose sensation of pain and heat. It is named as Boyle after its designer H Boyle, a British anesthesiologist.

BP APPARATUS

All fluids require some pressure to move from one point to another. More so when required to travel against the earth's gravity. Blood circulation occurs due to the hearts pressure in a living organism. This pressure of blood circulation can be high or low. This can be measured by using BP apparatus or sphygmomanometer.

BRONCHOFIBERSCOPE

It is a flexible bronchoscope utilizing fiber optics.

BRONCHOSCOPE

It is an instrument for inspecting the interior of the tracheobronchial tree and carrying out endobronchial diagnostic and therapeutic maneuvers such as taking specimens for culture and biopsy, and removing foreign bodies. These are usually rigid in nature.

C-ARM

C-arm units are so named because of their configuration. These radiographic units are used for fluoroscopic imaging during surgical, orthopedic, critical care, and emergency care procedures and also provide radiographic capabilities. It is especially used in imaging skeletal system.

COBALT TREATMENT EQUIPMENT

It is an equipment with radioactive cobalt-60 element, used in cancer therapy.

COLONOSCOPY

Endoscopic examination of the colon by transanally be means of fiberoptic endoscope.

COLPOSCOPE

A speculum for examining the vagina and cervix by means of magnifying lens.

COLOR DOPPLER

By the color Doppler, the color is superimposed on the anatomical gray-scale image. The flow of oxygenated and deoxygenated blood are differentiated by color.

CORONARY ANGIOGRAPH

A dye is injected into the patient's blood flow and it is photographed into a movie camera. The dye due to its higher density tries to move through constriction of coronary vessels when there should have been no constriction. This indicates thickening of vessels in the coronary cavities which supply blood to the heart muscles.

CT SCAN

The CT scanners are specifically designed for neuro- and radiological investigation with CT images. Radiologists could visualize easily (a) the ventricles of brain and (b) the repositions of the cerebrospinal fluid.

CYSTOSCOPE

This scope is used to visualize the bladder.

DEFIBRILLATOR

It is an apparatus which applies electrical impulses (shock) to the heart flow studies, especially for the blood flow in the human brain.

DOPPLER

Doppler also is an ultrasound machine but specifically used for blood flow studies, especially for the blood flow in the human brain.

ECHOCARDIOGRAPH (ECHO)

Echocardiograph is widely used and is a valuable instrument for carrying out cardiac examination and assessment of many congenital and acquired cardiac diseases.

ELECTROCARDIOGRAM (ECG)

Human heart functions on the basis of electrical signals produced on the muscle of body. These signals appear on the limbs and chest of a person. By taking these signals and representing them as wave forms, the physician can diagnose various diseases of the heart. Since these signals are electrical in nature it is called as electro cardiogram or cardiograph.

ELECTROENCEPHALOGRAPH (EEG)

Electroencephalograph is an instrument for recording the electrical activity of the brain by suitably placing surface electrodes on the scalp.

ELECTROMYOGRAPH (EMG)

Electromyograph is an instrument used for recording the electrical activity of the muscles to determine whether the muscles is active or not.

GAMMA KNIFE

It is an innovative radiation apparatus or tool which helps doctors in treating a number of brain disorders, brain tumors and other intracranial and vascular abnormalities with out opening the skull.

GASTROSCOPE

All endoscope for inspecting the interior of the stomach.

HOLTER MONITOR

It is an ambulatory ECG monitor, named after Holter, an American biophysicist. It is a portable continuous electrocardiographic recorder, typically monitoring two channels for 24 hours. It is used to detect the frequency and duration of cardiac rhythm, its disturbances and to assess pacemaker programing.

CLINICAL EQUIPMENT-LABORATORY

The laboratory provides many chemistries of the blood, urine and other human fluids such as saliva, gastric juices and semen. Lab also provides study of cells under magnification for variations in size, color and micro-organisms attacking human cells.

LAPAROSCOPY

It is an endoscopic equipment which makes the doctors to diagnose many conditions within the abdomen and pelvis. Laparoscope is a rigid telescope.

LASER EQUIPMENT

Laser is light amplification by stimulated emission of radiation. Laser equipment is a device that transfers a narrow beam of visible light into an extremely intense monochromatic small beam of radiation with high energies which is able to cut and dissolve tissue.

MAMMOGRAPHY

Female breast has lot of structures, and many variations occur during one's lifetime. Due to shape of the breasts and the tissues involved, regular X-ray machines can not be used to image them. The mammogram uses low power X-rays with convenient tube and X-ray plate between which the breast can be placed and X-rayed.

MONITOR

An apparatus used to observe or record specified data given as a series of events such as physiological signs as respiration, ECG, pulse rate blood pressure and temperature.

MAGNETIC RESONANCE IMAGING (MRI) SCAN

While X-rays under CT scan (X-ray) show bony structures and to some extent shades of other structures. MRI can reveal the cell structures and the changes. This is done by capturing human cell magnetic activity or to magnetic field produced by huge magnets (permanent) or electromagnets. The variations are imaged as pixels on a TV screen.

NEUROPHYSIOLOGY LABORATORY

In the laboratory of experimental neuromedicine, the investigation of the mechanisms underlying disturbances of cerebral cortex function in common neurological and neurosurgical diseases are being done, especially focus on post-traumatic or "lesional" epilepsy, as it shows a clear dysfunction of the cerebral cortex. More specifically, mainly study the interactions between the vascular system (especially the blood-brain barrier), astrocytes and neurons and their function under disease States. In the laboratory, the advanced brain imaging techniques as well as physiological recordings of brain activity are tested.

NUCLEAR SCAN

By injecting mild radioactive substances into blood stream, pictures can be captured by a nuclear camera (radioactive particles raise the electrical levels) and imaged on a TV screen. By studying these images many variations in the tissues can be detected.

OPHTHALMIC EXCIMER LASER

The word excimer is a contraction of the term exited dimer. Molecules made up of two identical atoms are called dimmers. In excimer lasers, we make use of two atoms—an inert gas and a halide specifically argon and fluoride. These two elements are in very small concentrations in a helium mixture known as premix. This laser with rare gas halides as a active medium whose beam is the ultraviolet spectrum and penetrates tissues only to a small distance and the beam breaks chemical bonds instead of generating heat to destroy the tissue. It is used in ophthalmological procedures.

POSITRON EMISSION TOMOGRAPHY (PET) SCAN

"PET" scanner, is a tomographic device that produces computerized cross sectional images of biochemical activity in the brain or other organs through the use of radioactive tracers.

PHYSIOLOGICAL LABORATORY

The physiological laboratory provides electrophysiological activity of organs which can be trapped from the surface of the human body. An example of the organ is heart/brain. The laboratory provides not only wave form but other variable, such as amplitude duration, and trend. These are mainly used with cath lab or cardiothoracic department.

PULMONARY FUNCTION TEST (PFT)

Pulmonary function test provides, a means for automated clinical procedures and analysis technique for carrying out a complete evaluation of the lung function of the respiratory process.

PULMONARY AID

Pulmonary aid provides fine mist of dilated medication directly into the lungs. By doing so, the constriction in the lungs can be lessened and patient can be returned to normal breathing from asthmatic condition. The machine incorporates a pressure pump and a nebulizer (a pin hole through which fluids are sent at a pressures).

PULSE OXIMETER

Pulse oximeter refers to the determination of the percentage of the oxygen saturation in the circulating arterial blood.

SIGMOIDOSCOPY

This refers to the direct examination of the interior of sigmoid colon.

TREADMILL

Treadmill is used to make the patient to walk briskly during ECG testing. By comparing ECG at rest and ECG during exercise, various condition of the heart can be studied.

ULTRASOUND

Ultrasound is used for imaging the structure inside the body with sound waves of extremely high frequency (above 20,000 Hz inaudible to the human ear).

URETERORENOSCOPY

Ureterorenosocpy is visualizing the interior of the ureter and kidney by means of fiberoptic endoscope for taking biopsy, removal or crushing of stones, etc.

VENTILATOR

The Ventilator is a device which mechanically assists patients who are unable to breath with oxygen and air, and sometimes it is referred to as artificial respiration.

X-RAYS

X-rays are electromagnetic radiations similar to light but shorter in wave length and capable of penetrating solids. It was discovered by Wilhelm Rontgen, a German physicist.

In addition to the above equipments, there are nebulizer, suction machine, infusion pump, syringe pump, surgical diathermy, heart lung machine, laryngoscope, gastroscopy, incubator C pap, bipap, cryopump and other hundreds of equipments which are used in laboratory, ICU, IMCU, OT, etc.

Some of the above mentioned equipments are life saving equipments and some of them are used for diagnostic purpose in patient care. Some equipments are used for monitoring the vital parameters of the patients which help in deciding on patient treatment. For example, blood reports or scan reports which are generated by the medical equipments are very important for treating doctor to treat or change the line of treatment to patient. Since these equipments are essential, hospitals keep equipping themselves with latest machines for patient care. However, for purchase of any equipments, the technical sanction, financial sanction and the administrative sanction from the respective departments are required.

Since equipment are very expensive, under utilization may lead to loss to the hospital. Hence, the proposal for purchasing the equipment should come from the technical department or the department concerned. Based on the quotation, the top management sanctions the amount if the equipment is necessary and viable.

Cooperation and coordination among the top level managers, interest and involvement of biomedical engineer helps in purchase of medical equipments in many hospitals. The purchase procedure depends on the hospital policy

1. Hospital should have a clear policy regarding:
   a. Criteria for purchase
   b. Procedure for purchase
   c. Sale of equipment
   d. Condemning equipment
   e. Transfer or shifting of equipment, etc.

2. After the purchase, qualified biomedical engineers are appointed to look after the equipment.

DUTIES AND RESPONSIBILITIES OF BIOMEDICAL ENGINEERS

1. Purchasing quality equipments from the authorized dealers and the distributors
2. Collecting quotations and comparing the price, quality, running cost/ recurring cost of the equipment, cost of spares
3. Following up with suppliers for after sales service
4. Periodical calliberation of the equipment
5. Maintaining data regarding availability of spares and cost of spares
6. Insuring the equipment if not covered
7. Calculating the cost of AMC or CAMS
8. Maintaining a register for meantime for break down or meantime to repair of the particular equipment
9. Collecting the schematic drawings and equipment specification at the time of purchase
10. Maintaining inventory of the equipments
11. Maintaining register showing new purchases and condemned items
12. Maintaining record of equipment wise break down details
13. Maintain an inventory register with transfers or shifting of equipment from one ward to other ward or unit
14. Entering sale of equipment properly in accounts books and stock registers
15. Keeping a unique number for every equipment, which reveals the location, department, type of equipment and the serial number of that particular equipment.

The important key indicator for biomedical engineering department is to minimize the break down calls by preventive maintenance and reduce the meantime to repair the equipments.

EQUIPMENTS REQUIRED FOR ICU, OT, TRIAGE, AND CLINICAL LABORATORY

1. High quality multi parameter monitors
2. BP apparatus
3. Nebulizer
4. Syringe pump
5. Infusion pump
6. Alpha/water beds

7. 12 lead ECG recorders
8. Electrical vaccum machine
9. Focus light
10. Needle destroyer
11. Thermometer
12. Laryngoscope
13. Stethoscope
14. Ambu bag
15. X-ray lobby
16. Fumigator
17. Defibrillator
18. Ventilators with or without compressure
19. C PAP
20. BIPAP
21. External pacemaker
22. Dialysis machine
23. O_2 line
24. Compressed air.

OPERATION THEATER

1. OT table (electrohydraulic with remote)
2. OT light (dual dome, with a minimum of 1,10,000 + 1,10,000 lux and shadowless)
3. Pendants (for O_2, N_2O, compressed air, vaccum outlets)
4. Multiparameter monitor (ECG, SPO_2, NIBA, EL-CO_2, temperature)
5. Syringe pumps
6. BP apparatus
7. Nebulizer
8. Electrical vaccum machine
9. Needle destroyer
10. Ambu bag
11. Thermometer
12. Laryngoscope
13. Stethoscope
14. X-ray lobby
15. Fumigator
16. Boyles apparatus with circle absorber, soda lime canister, vaporizer
17. Anesthesia ventilator
18. Surgical diathermy

19. Defibrillator
20. Heart lung machine (in cardiac thoracic OT)
21. Microscopic (for neurosurgeries).

Any other equipment required for special surgeries.

CLINICAL LABORATORY

Histopathology laboratory

1. Tissue processor
2. Embed or machine
3. Water bath
4. Microtone
5. Slide stainer
6. Heating unit for melting wax
7. Incubator
8. Hot air oven
9. Microwave
10. Centrifuge
11. Binocular microscope
12. Refrigerator.

Clinical pathology

1. Urine analyzer
2. Semen analyzer
3. Centrifuge
4. Microscope
5. Fluorescence microscope
6. Refrigerator

BIOCHEMISTRY LABORATORY

1. Autoanalyzer
2. Semiautoanalyzer
3. Electrolyte machine
4. Proton
5. Immulite machine
6. Immunofixation
7. Radioimmunoacid machine
8. Blood cell counter
9. QBC centrifuge with reader
10. Spectrophotometer
11. Prothrombin analyzer
12. Urine analyzer
13. Centrifuge
14. Microscope
15. Incubator
16. Water bath
17. Desk top sterilizer.

EQUIPMENTS REQUIRED FOR PHYSIOTHERAPY DEPARTMENT

I. Therapeutic equipments

1. Short wave therapy equipment
2. Microwave therapy equipment
3. Ultrasound wave therapy equipment
4. Longwave therapy equipment
5. Laser therapy equipment
6. Tread mill
7. Cryotherapy equipment
8. Various exercise equipments.

II. Diagnostic

1. EMG
2. Manual muscle testing equipments
3. Nerve stimulation test equipment.

CHAPTER 17

Biomedical Waste Management

An important area in which the top management of a hospital should concentrate is the disposal of biomedical waste.

It is a statutory requirement for any hospital to get a license/approval from the State Pollution Control Board for proper disposal of biomedical waste generated in various departments of the hospital like the following:

1. Wards
2. Investigation departments
3. Canteen
4. Operation theaters
5. Dressing department
6. ICU, IMCU, casualty, labor room and others.

Biomedical waste include clinical waste like gauze, cotton: Used sharp needles/blades syringes, aerosol cans, syringes, plastic bottles (noninfected), containers (infected), etc.

Steps in disposing biomedical waste collection:

The first step involves collecting the waste by the ward nursing staff, paramedicals, house keeping boys and staff working in various departments. They ensure that the various color code bins are to segregate different types of biomedical waste.

This biomedical waste is collected regularly by concerned person in appropriate color plastic covers or bins and is taken to the central segregation place.

Disposal of biomedical waste are discussed below:

SEGREGATION AND COLLECTION

Since disposal of waste generated from the hospital is an important statutory requirement, care is to be taken at every stage. In every ward and department, color code bins are used to segregate the waste based on plastic, needles, bio-disposable items etc. The staff must strictly adhere to the color code from the very beginning. This waste is collected and taken to the central segregation place, in separate color bags for easy identification and segregation. Each bag is given a label with time and date along with the name of the department. These bags are securely tied and are stored in an area not accessible to the public and also safe from rodents, insects, etc.

DISPOSAL

Precaution in handling and disposal of clinical sharps.

Disposal of clinical/hospital waste:
Since clinical sharp are for single use, the user must discard them after use directly into a sharp container, without leaving them lying around. The sharp containers are also labeled, the aperture is tightly closed to prevent spillage or tampering. They should be carried by the handle without holding them close to the body. The items should not be retrieved and pressed down. The container is locked using the closure mechanism, when it is full. In case, if sharps spill from a container they should be retrieved by using personal protective equipment (PPE) like gloves, mask, etc.

COLOR CODIFICATION OF BIOMEDICAL WASTE

Red—Blood sets, catheters, gloves, IV sets, plastic bottles, ryles tubes, syringes, urobages.

Yellow—Infectious waste/cotton/gauzes/blood strained cotton/pads/underpads.

Blue—Unbroken IV glass bottles, syrup bottles, vials, other glass items.

Green—Cardboards, fruits, leaves, paper items, tea cups, other food items.

White Jars—Ampoules, blades, broken items. The jar containing 1% sodium hypochlorite solutions.

In addition to ward in-charge nurses, the floor managers and heads of the departments are also responsible for waste identification and segregation.

The hospital infection control team is responsible for assuring policy and guidance on the safe handling, storage, segregation and disposal of clinical waste and it is reviewed regularly. They are also responsible for identifying resources to ensure adequate training and proper equipments are available. They have to maintain records, documentation of the training given to show during inspection.

CHAPTER 18

Medical Ethics

Medical ethics is a system of moral principles that apply values and judgments to the practice of medicine.

BASIC PRINCIPLES OF MEDICAL ETHICS

The most important ethical principles that one need to know in clinical practice are outlined below. They will help and guide to ethical decision-making.

Autonomy—This ethical value refers to the ability of the competent patient to make his/her own decisions about choosing or refusing treatments.

Beneficence—Another major principle of medical ethics that refers to the actions taken by a medical professional that are considered to be in the best interests of the patient. This ethical value is sometimes in conflict with the autonomy of the patient. The physician may feel that a certain treatment is necessary for the patient's wellbeing, but the patient denies the advised treatment. This actually comes up rather frequently in practice. Usually the patient's autonomy wins out, assuming the patient is mentally competent and understands the pros and cons of the proposed treatment. If mental competency is in question, occasionally a psychiatric and/or neurologic evaluation may be required to determine the patient's ability to make appropriate medical decisions.

Non-maleficence (*primum non nocere*, "first, do no harm")—This is a long-standing dictum in medical ethics–that it is better to do no harm to the patient than to do them good. This comes into play many times a day in medical practice. One needs to know the likelihood of whether a certain medication or other treatment will cause harm compared to the likelihood that it will be beneficial. Physicians are constantly making these kinds of decisions using the so-called risk/benefit ratio, which is often a matter of judgment and experience, but also requires knowledge of the medical literature on the subject. In fact the medical literature can certainly be helpful in these situations and can provide support for the decisions that one make.

Unfortunately, there are many situations in medicine where this type of knowledge has not yet been obtained or the results of studies are not clear. The physician must then discuss the options carefully and clearly to the patient and the family, obtain whatever consultants that may help in the decision-making process and together arrive at a consensus on the best course of action.

Double effect—a corollary to the non-maleficence principle of medical ethics whereby the positive effect of a treatment may also cause harm at the same time. The best example of this is in the field of palliative care in which a patient suffering from pain or shortness of breath due to an incurable terminal disease might be prescribed morphine to help control the suffering, even knowing that death may be hastened by suppressing the respiratory drive as a side effect of the morphine. In this case, alleviating the extreme suffering is felt to be beneficial to the alternative of being miserable during the last hours of an inevitable death.

OTHER MEDICAL ETHICAL GUIDELINES

Informed Consent—This medical ethical guideline basically relates to the autonomy of the patient to choose or decline a medical procedure or a potentially harmful test or treatment. A form presented to the patient or to the family surrogate, if the patient is incapacitated and unable to sign, which, if signed, indicates that permission is given by the patient to go ahead with the procedure and that the patient has full knowledge of the potential risks. Informed consent should be administered by the primary doctor or consultant anesthetist performing the procedure.

Confidentiality, or patient-physician privilege, is a medical ethical value mandated in this country by the privacy rule or better known as Health Insurance Portability and Accountability Act (HIPAA) laws. These are a rather rigid set of rules that does help protect the patient's privacy, but are sometimes very frustrating to family members because no one will tell them what is going on with their loved one in the hospital. This often results in poor communication and ultimately anger developing in family members. This puts more onus on the physician to be sure to discuss the patient's condition with family members, assuming he has the patient's verbal permission to do so.

Certain laws provide for specific exceptions to the patient-physician privilege, requiring physicians to report sexually transmitted diseases, gunshot wounds, impaired drivers, underage abortions, etc.

Telling the truth to a patient about the diagnosis is sometimes a medical ethical issue in certain cultures. In America, people usually feel it is important for the patient to know what is wrong with him/her. They usually know anyway that something awful is happening. To have the diagnosis withheld can create greater stress and anxiety than knowing what it is and dealing directly with it.

Conflicts of interest—There are many different conflicts of interest that may occur in medical practice. Sometimes it is difficult to draw the line between what is acceptable, which is medically ethical and what is not. For example, a physician who sees a patient with palpitations may wish to do an investigation for which the doctor receives additional reimbursement. This is generally considered acceptable, even though it may be construed as a conflict of interest. If the doctor refers the patient for an investigation to an outpatient testing facility of which s/he is part owner, this is taboo and tantamount to fraud.

Despite these nuances, the main intent of this medical ethics principle is that a physician should never allow financial interests or other nonmedical interests to interfere with or influence medical judgment in the care of patients. The same principle applies to avoiding relationships with pharmaceutical companies that may potentially influence what medication you may give to a patient.

Sexual relationships with patients or family members of patients are considered highly unethical and may result in loss of license or prosecution.

Medical treatment of family members is somewhat controversial and not completely prohibited although generally not felt to be a good idea, particularly for major medical problems or surgery. The prescribing of narcotics to a family member is much more strictly prohibited and will likely lead to some retribution.

Medical futility (nonbeneficial care) is a term indicating that the patient is so seriously ill that if the heart stops or if respirations cease, providing extraordinary resuscitative measures like cardiopulmonary resuscitation and/or artificial ventilation will not provide any benefit for the patient whose death is imminent anyway with or without the treatment.

This is an extremely difficult medical ethical issue for many families to grapple with. If the family has to make this decision, there may be a certain amount of guilt that will be carried long after the patient has expired. If a patient has an advanced directive that clearly states his/her wishes in this regard, this takes the pressure off the family to decide.

If the patient does not have an advanced directive and if the patient is unable to answer the questions about CPR, and if the family cannot or does not want to decide, the physician *can* legally make the decision, in some if not most States, that CPR or ventilator treatment would be medically futile and not warranted. Most of the time, however, it would be beneficial if the family were in agreement with the physician's decision on this. In fact, many physicians do not want to make that call without clear family support for two reasons: No matter how difficult it is, families want to be involved in these discussions, and also because of potential medico-legal issues that may occur if the family does not agree with the doctor's decision.

Reproductive medicine—This is becoming a greater medical ethical issue every day as we develop better ways to "create" pregnancies in those who would have been incapable of this otherwise. Where does one draw the line on who gets how many children?

Religious beliefs—Medical ethical issues such as abortion and stem cell research are very emotional concerns that reach to the very core of morality and are closely intertwined with religious beliefs of millions of people around the world. Standards and policies regarding these issues are not easily made and are subject to change because there are so many people who feel strongly about one side or the other. Physicians and pharmacists sometimes get caught in the middle because of their own religious beliefs which may be in opposition to their patients' wishes or to government regulations.

Medical research—There are clear guidelines followed by the medical research community about what is medically ethical research and what is not. There are indeed many medical questions that will yet to answer because research required to find out would be unethical. Thankfully, these guidelines on human experimentation are known worldwide now because of the Declaration of Helsinki developed by the World Medical Association. In India, schedule 'y' of ICMR and good clinical practice [GLP] are followed.

Utilization of resources—This will likely prove to be one of the most important medical ethical issues of the not too distant future as medical costs continue to skyrocket and medical resources become more limited. The specific issues to be decided will include things like whether an 80-year-old person will be able to have insurance to cover the costs of chemotherapy for cancer, or hemodialysis for end-stage renal disease, or prolonged ICU care for respiratory failure. These are issues that cannot be decided very easily.

Medical ethical issues are an important part of clinical practice. One will almost certainly be faced with some difficult ethical dilemmas at some time or another. One's knowledge and experience will help him decide along with close communication with family members and consultants. Ethics committees and palliative care teams are sometimes available to help with such problems as well. In a difficult situation, you should use whatever resources are available to help in the process. Do not try to "go it alone" unless there is no choice in the matter.

IMPORTANCE OF COMMUNICATION

Many ethical conflicts in medical ethics are traceable back to a lack of communication. Communication breakdowns between patients and their healthcare team, between family members, or between members of the medical community, can all lead to disagreements and strong feelings. These breakdowns should be remedied and many apparently insurmountable ethical problems can be solved with open lines of communication.

CHAPTER 19

Medicolegal Issues

Medicolegal cases (MLCs) are an integral part of medical practice that is frequently encountered by medical officers (MO). Proper handling, an accurate documentation of these cases is of prime importance to avoid legal complications.

All medical officers working in hospitals/field medical units/non medical units encounter medicolegal issues which should be handled in accordance with the law of the land.

Since law and order is a state subject, there are differences in the legal procedures being followed by different States. Medical officers should acquaint themselves with medicolegal procedures that are in vogue in the state in which they are serving.

DEFINITION OF MLCs IN MEDICAL PRACTICE

A MLC is defined as "any case of injury or ailment where, the attending doctor after history taking and clinical examination considers that investigations by law enforcement agencies are warranted to ascertain circumstances and fix responsibility regarding the said injury or ailment according to the law".

Who will Label a Case as MLC

a. RMO/Casualty Medical Officer/MO in-charge of Medical Inspection (MI) room Duty Medical Officer (DMO)/MO in-charge ward who is attending to the case, may label a case as a MLC.
b. The decision to label a case as MLC should be based on sound professional judgment, after a detailed history taking and thorough clinical examination.

EXAMPLES OF MLCs

The following are some of the examples of MLCs and Medical Officers should use their professional judgment to decide any other cases not enumerated in the list:

a. Assault and battery, including domestic violence and child abuse.
b. Accidents like Road Traffic Accidents (RTA), industrial accidents, etc.
c. Cases of trauma with suspicion of foul play.
d. Electrical injuries.
e. Poisoning, alcohol intoxication.
f. Undiagnosed coma.
g. Chemical injuries.
h. Burns and scalds.
i. Sexual offences.
j. Criminal abortions.
k. Attempted suicide.
l. Cases of asphyxia as a result of hanging, strangulation, drowning, suffocation, etc.
m. Custodial deaths.
n. Death in the operation theater.
o. Unnatural deaths.
p. Death due to snake bite or animal bite.
q. Fire arm injuries.
r. Drug overdose.
s. Drug abuse.
t. Dead brought to the accident and emergency dept/MI room (found dead) and deaths occurring within 24 hours of hospitalization without establishment of a diagnosis.

GENERAL GUIDELINES FOR DEALING WITH MEDICOLEGAL CASES

In emergencies, resuscitation and stabilization of the patient will be carried out first and medico legal formalities may be completed subsequently. The consent for treatment is implied in all emergencies.

Emergency medical care will be administered to all cases brought to any hospital irrespective of their entitlement. In non-entitled cases, after the initial stabilization, the patient may be transferred to the nearest government hospital, and if necessary by service ambulance.

Cases of trauma will be labeled as MLCs, if there is a suspicion of foul play, even if the incident is not of recent origin.

All MI rooms and hospitals will maintain a MLC register and the MLC will be initiated and documented in the register. Personal particulars, identification marks, finger prints of the individual will be noted. Particulars of the person accompanying the patient will also be noted.

Medicolegal documents should be prepared in duplicate, with utmost care giving all necessary details, preferably written with a ball-point pen and avoiding overwriting. If any overwriting or correction is made, it should be authenticated with the full signature and stamp of the MO. Abbreviations should be avoided.

Senior registrar and equivalent in the hospitals should be immediately informed as and when a MLC is registered or admitted. The particulars of the patient and a short summary of the case should be mentioned in the DMO report book.

Nearest of the kin should be informed if the address is available. The police should be informed. Under Section 39 of Criminal Procedure Code, the attending MO is legally bound to inform the police about the arrival of a MLC. Any failure to report the occurrence of a MLC may invite prosecution under Sections 176 and/or 202 of IPC. Simultaneously the verbal communication should invariably be followed by communication in writing subsequently.

In case of discharge/transfer/death of such a case in the hospital, the police should be informed.

Medicolegal documents should be considered as confidential records and should be stored under safe custody to avoid tampering. Medical records must be thorough, complete and should document each and every significant event in the course of care of the patient. All the documents including case sheets, X-rays and investigation reports will be preserved meticulously in the medical record section indefinitely and handed over to the concerned authorities (police investigating officer/court/court of inquiry) as and when required.

Prompt attention, correct triage and safe transfer of a patient from one facility to another as required should be carried out in all cases and not delayed because of the medicolegal nature of the case.

Opinion on severity of injuries should be given after the X-ray reports are received in cases of injury to bones/joints.

Samples and specimens collected for medicolegal purposes will be properly sealed, labeled and handed over to the investigating officer detailed by the police. CMO of the hospital will have to ensure that the documents are kept in the custody of an appropriate officer till the case is finally decided or cleared by the police and judicial authorities.

Dying declaration: In cases where the patient wishes to make a dying declaration, the magistrate will be intimated. If the magistrate is unable to come and record a statement or where the MO feels that he might not be able to reach the patient in time, the MO may record the dying declaration himself in presence of two independent witnesses whose signatures have to be affixed in the document. The MO should certify the soundness of mind of the person making the dying declaration.

Battle casualties (BC) and battle accidents (BA) are not to be reported as MLCs. The medical cause of death in these cases may however be certified by the RMO.

If a death has been reported by the hospital authorities as medicolegal and is decided otherwise by the police after investigation, a certificate to that effect is required to be obtained from the investigating officer in the format attached as Enclosure 1, along with a copy of the Panchanama when the body is returned to the hospital.

PRECAUTIONS TO BE TAKEN IN MLCs

a. The complete available particulars of the patient should be noted down along with two identification marks. Particulars of the person accompanying the patient will also be noted down.
b. One should not rely on memory while writing reports or during recording of evidence in a court of law.
c. Complicated cases should be discussed with seniors and colleagues.
d. No cause of death should be mentioned in the death certificate. The statement that "exact cause is to be ascertained by postmortem examination" is to be endorsed.
e. In MLCs, the body will not be handed over to the NOK/relatives. The civil police will be informed and the body handed over to them. The police will, after the medicolegal formalities, handover the body to the NOK/relatives.
f. Death of a service person, in an accident involving a military aircraft will not be reported as an MLC to the civil police. The enquiry conducted by the competent military authorities will suffice.
g. An MLC should be reported by the first health care establishment in which the individual is received. In cases where a patient has been transferred before initiation of a report, the hospital to which he is transferred can initiate the report. It is important to ensure that the medical records are comprehensive before a patient is transferred. The fact as to whether or not medicolegal formalities have been initiated should invariably be mentioned in the transfer notes.

GUIDELINES FOR PRESERVATION OF MEDICOLEGAL EVIDENCE

a. Medicolegal evidence should be preserved and subsequently sent or handed over to the investigating authorities for forensic examination and production as evidence in a court of law. All evidences will be identified, sealed and labeled properly. They will be kept in safe custody and handed over to the investigating officer of the case. Once collected, loss/destruction of evidence is a punishable offence. Failure to collect, destruction or loss of such an exhibit is punishable under Sec 201 of IPC.

b. The evidence required to be preserved is related to the nature of a case. In injury cases, the following articles should be preserved in sealed envelopes:
   i. Clothing worn by the patient showing evidence of injury such as tears, bullet holes, cuts, blood stains, etc.
   ii. In case of multiple tears, cuts or holes, etc. each piece of evidence should be encircled and numbered with matching description in the MLC report and case sheet.
   iii. Bullets recovered from a body should be marked by etching an initial or a mark on the bottom before preservation.
   iv. All evidence collected should be mentioned in medicolegal documents to establish the chain of custody in a court of law subsequently.

c. In cases of suspected poisoning the following articles should be preserved and ensured that they are forwarded for forensic examination:
   i. Gastric lavage/gastric contents/vomitus and soiled clothing
   ii. Blood, urine and any other relevant body fluid depending on the poison ingested.

d. In cases of burns and carbon monoxide poisoning, the following articles should be preserved in sealed envelopes:
   i. Articles soiled with inflammable substances like burnt pieces of clothing, scalp hair, etc.
   ii. Blood (and not serum) for carbon monoxide levels.

e. In sexual offences, the following articles should be preserved in sealed envelopes:
   i. Clothing worn by the patient and showing evidence of blood stains or seminal stains, stains of mud, tears/cuts, etc.
   ii. Vaginal swab preferably from posterior fornix/anal swab.

GUIDELINES FOR PRESERVATION OF MEDICOLEGAL DOCUMENTS

a. Original copies of all medicolegal documents should be produced whenever asked for in a court of law.
b. All original copies of certificates and reports issued for medicolegal purposes are to be preserved till the finalization of case in the court of law.
c. Documents pertaining to admitted fatal MLCs are to be processed and preserved as laid down in concerned policy letters.

SPECIAL PRECAUTIONS IN CASES OF DEATH IN THE HOSPITAL

a. It should be ensured that proper packing is done before transferring the dead body to the mortuary.
b. The mortuary staff should note down two identification marks of the deceased and confirm the particulars of the deceased as noted on the metal identification disk on the right great toe of the deceased by checking with the accompanying documents.
c. Willingness/unwillingness certificate for autopsy and body handing taking over certificate should be obtained.

GENERAL GUIDELINES FOR SUDDEN DEATH/FOUND DEAD CASES

a. Deaths, which require medicolegal investigation, may be divided into three main groups:
   i. Deaths either known or suspected to have been caused by unnatural causes.
   ii. Sudden death cause unknown.
   iii. Found dead—unattended death.
b. As per ICD 10, "sudden death cause unknown" could be as follows:
   i. Instantaneous death.
   ii. Death occurring less than 24 hours from onset of symptoms, not otherwise explained.
   iii. Death in circumstances where the body of the deceased was found and no cause could be discovered. Found dead.
   iv. Death not otherwise specified (NOS). Unknown cause of mortality.

c. Deaths due to natural causes fall within the medicolegal domain when they occur in custody, clashes, accidents and sometimes even during violent arguments. Therefore, a medical officer should not certify the cause of death in such cases without holding a post mortem examination, even if there is strong evidence of the underlying cause.
d. The deceased should be examined in detail by attending MO and resuscitation will be attempted, failing which death will be confirmed
e. Two identification marks should be noted.
f. Circumstances leading to death should be ascertained from person bringing and identifying the body.
g. All particulars and address of the person(s) bringing the deceased should be noted in the case sheet and history given by them will be endorsed in the case sheet as alleged history.
h. Civil Police is to be informed in writing with copies to all concerned.
i. Body should be handed over to civil police for further disposal. Under no circumstances should the body be handed over to next of kin directly. Alternately clearance in writing should be obtained from civil police for disposal of the body.
j. In case the body is being sent for medicolegal autopsy to other hospital, brief summary of the case should be given to civil police.
k. A receipt for handing over the body to police should be taken and kept along with the case documents.
l. The following documents should be initiated:
   i. Admission flimsy
   ii. Case sheet
   iii. Death certificate
   iv. Record of summary in the medicolegal case register
   v. Dead body handing taking over certificate.

MEDICOLEGAL ASPECTS OF SEXUAL OFFENCES

Victims of alleged sexual offences like rape may be brought to the MI room or may come on their own. In the event the victim comes directly, the civil police will be informed and necessary action should be taken to register a case. The examination may be carried out at a center authorized for medicolegal work with forensic experts. Where the examination is carried out by a service MO, it should preferably be done by a lady MO or gynecologist or by MO i/c MI room in the presence of a female attendant. In cases of sodomy, the victim may be examined by the MO i/c MI room.

MEDICOLEGAL ASPECTS OF POISONING

a. Poison may be defined as any substance which when absorbed into the body or by local action on the tissues injures health or destroys life.

b. Medicolegal aspects of poisons.

   Sections 284, 299, 300, 304A, 324, 326 and 328 of IPC deal with offences relating to handling and administration of poisonous substances. As per Indian law, administration of any substance with the intention of causing hurt or death is punishable.

c. Guidelines in case of poisoning

   i. When poisoning is suspected, every attempt must be made to save the patient's life. The patient shall be shifted immediately to the hospital/MI room nearby.
   ii. Case sheet shall be initiated, noting personal particulars of the victim, along with date and time of reporting. The particulars of the person accompanying the patient should also be noted.
   iii. The victim should be protected from further exposure of poisoning but no clothing shall be thrown away, as they might be useful for chemical analysis.
   iv. MLC should be initiated after filling the MLC register available at MI Room.
   v. The patient will be admitted if the medical condition is serious.
   vi. Civil police must be informed.
   vii. The treating doctor/authorized nursing staff will only be permitted to administer food and medicines to the patient.
   viii. A careful history is to be elicited including the relationship of food or medicine taken and the toxic manifestations. All signs and symptoms are to be noted carefully.
   ix. The vomitus, urine, feces, stomach wash, sample of food or medicine taken should be preserved in a sterile bottle. Any suspicious bottle or utensil seen near the victim, the clothes and bed clothes used last by the victim are all to be preserved for chemical analysis. Suitable preservatives may be used for these purposes depending upon the nature of the sample. The name and concentration of preservative used should invariably be mentioned in the label and/or accompanying documents.
   x. It is advisable to take the second opinion and advice of a senior professional colleague in all matters regarding diagnosis and treatment. Use of poison information services may also be made.

xi. If there is any indication of danger to the general public, for example, food poisoning from a hotel, the public health authorities must be notified at once so that suitable remedial measures are taken.

xii. In case of food poisoning from unit cookhouse, the DMO has to inform the incident to administrative authorities.

xiii Where required, a magistrate should be called to take down the dying declaration.

xiv. Medical certification and cause of death will be issued with mention that 'cause of death to be ascertained after chemical analysis'.

xv. Various samples of medicolegal importance should be preserved and handed over to the police for forensic examination.

xvi. A receipt shall be obtained from the police for all samples that are handed over for forensic examination.

GUIDELINES FOR ACTION IN CASE A PATIENT IS FOUND MISSING FROM THE HOSPITAL

a. When a patient is reported missing from the hospital, all efforts will first be made by the hospital to locate him/her. Information will be sent to the unit, station HQ, CMP, civil police and NOK regarding his/her absence from the hospital. When all efforts to locate the patient do not succeed, he/she should be discharged in absentia.

b. After being discharged in absentia, if the patient reports again to the hospital, he/ she should be readmitted for further treatment, if required. The period of absence from the hospital should be reported to the hospital authorities and it should be mentioned in the case sheet.

CONCLUSION

The way in which medicolegal issues are handled has a profound impact on the public image of the Hospitals. Therefore, MLCs must be handled tactfully by the MOs. The administrative authorities must also help in maintaining goodwill and avoiding legal complications.

CHAPTER 20

Consumer Protection Act, 1986 and Hospitals

With the development of interest of the society to protect the interests of the consumer, the consumer protection act, 1986 is a significant development in the shape of providing the redressal machinery for settling the consumer disputes in a convenient, inexpensive, effective and speedy way.

The Act provides for district forums, state commissions and the national commission which can be approached not only by the individual consumer himself but also by any recognized voluntary consumer association on his behalf.

EXTENT AND COVERAGE OF THE ACT

The salient features of the act are summed up as under:

- The Act applies to all goods and services unless specifically exempted by the central government
- It covers all the sectors whether private, public or cooperative
- The provisions of the Act are compensatory in nature
- The provisions of this Act are in addition to and not in derogation of the provisions of any other law for the time being in force.

COMPLAINANT

This chapter defines every area under the concept of treating the patient as a consumer.

Any allegation, in writing made by a complaint that the service hired or availed of or agreed to be hired or availed of by him suffer from deficiency in any respect.

CONSUMER

Any "person" who hires or avils of any services for a consideration which has been paid or promised or partly paid and partly promised any include any beneficiary of such services for consideration paid or promised, or partly paid and partly promised, or under any system of deferred payment, when such services are availed of with the approval of the first mentioned person.

- A person who receives medical treatment in Government or Charitable Hospital, which provides treatment to one and all free of cost, is not a consumer under the Act.
- A person who receives treatment in a Government or charitable hospital which provides treatment free of cost to some and on consideration to some would be a consumer, even if he has not paid any fees.
- In case of death of patient who is a consumer, legal heirs (representatives), of the deceased will be considered as "consumer". If the payment has been made by any person who is not a legal heir of the deceased he too will considered as 'consumer'.

FEES/PAYMENT

Fees may have been fully paid in cash or cheques, or undertaking that it will be paid, which is accepted by the doctor/hospital. The fees may have been given partly (as advance) with the understanding that the remaining bill will be paid subsequently. The payment may be done by the patient himself or by someone else for the patient, e.g. father for child, or the husband for wife.

The three words used above (deficiency, person, and service) explained under this Act are as follows:

DEFICIENCY

Deficiency means any fault, imperfection, shortcoming or inadequacy in the quality, nature and manner of performance which is required to be maintained by or under any law for the time being in force or has been undertaken to be performed by a person in pursuance of a contract or otherwise in relation to any service.

PERSON

Person includes the following:

1. A firm whether registered or not
2. A Hindu undivided family

3. A cooperative society
4. Every other association of persons whether registered under the Societies Registration Act, 1860, or not.

SERVICE

Service includes the provision of facilities in connection with banking, financing, insurance, transport, processing, supply of electrical or other energy, board or lodging or both, housing construction, entertainment, amusement or the purveying of news or other information but does not include the rendering of any service free of charge or under a contract of personal services.

THE ACT WITH RELATION TO THE HOSPITALS OR MEDICAL PROFESSION

On the meaning of the word "service" in relation to medical profession, the Supreme Court in Indian Medical Association VVP Shantha and Ors (Supra) came to the following conclusions:

- Service rendered to a patient by a medical practitioner (except where the doctor rendered service free of charge to every patient or under a contract of personal service), by way consultation, diagnosis and treatment, both medicinal and surgical, would fall within the ambit of 'service' as defined in section 2(1) (o) of the Act.
- The expression 'contract of personal service' in section 2(1) (o) of the Act cannot be confined to contracts for employment of domestic servants only and the said expression would include the employment of a medical officer for the purpose of rendering medical service to the employer. The service rendered by a medical officer to his employer under the contract of employment would be outside the purview of 'service' as defined in section 2(1) (o) of the Act.
- Service rendered at a government hospital/health center/dispensary or at non-government hospital/nursing home where no charge whatsoever is made from any person availing the service and all patients (rich and poor) are given free service—is outside the purview of the expression "service" as defined in section 2(1) (o) of the Act. The payment of a token amount for registration purpose only at the hospital/nursing home would not alter the position.
- Service rendered at a non-government hospital/nursing home where charges are required to be paid by the person availing such services falls within the purview of the expression 'service' as defined in section 2(1) (o) of the Act.

- Service rendered at government hospital/health center/dispensary or at an non-government nursing home where charges are required to be paid by persons who are in a position to pay and persons who cannot afford to pay are rendered service free of charge would fall within the ambit of the expression 'service' as defined in section 2(1) (o) of the Act irrespective of the fact that the service is rendered free of charge to persons who are not in a position to pay for such services. Free service, by such doctors and hospitals would also be 'service' and the recipient a 'consumer' under the Act.
- Service rendered by a medical or hospital/nursing home cannot be regarded as service rendered free of charge, if the persons availing the service has taken an insurance policy for medical care where under the policy charges for consultation diagnosis and medical treatment are borne by the insurance company and such service would fall within the ambit of 'service' as defined in section 2(1) (o) of the Act.
- Similarly, when as a part of the conditions of service, the employer bears the expenses of medical treatment of an employee and his family member dependent on him, the service rendered to such an employee and his family members by a medical practitioner or a hospital/nursing home would not be free of charge and would constitute 'service' under section 2(1) (o) of the Act.

It has included the following categories of doctors/hospitals under this Section:

1. All medical/dental practitioners doing independent medical/dental practice unless rendering only free service.
2. Private hospitals charging all patients.
3. All hospitals having free as well as paying patients and all the paying and free category patients receiving treatment in such hospitals.
4. Medical/dental practitioners and hospitals paid by an insurance firm for the treatment of a client or an employment for that of an employee.

It exempts only those hospitals and the medical/dental practitioners of such hospitals which offer free service to all patients.

Further, this judgment concedes that the summary procedure prescribed by the CPA would suit only glaring cases of negligence and in complaints involving complicated issues requiring recording of the evidence of experts, the complainant can be asked to approach the civil courts.

Also, this judgment says that the deficiency in service means only negligence in a medical negligence case and it would be determined under CPA by applying the same test as is applied in an action for damages for negligence in a civil court.

As a result of this judgment, virtually all private and government hospitals and the doctors employed by them and the independent medical/dental practitioners except primary health centers, birth control measures, anti malaria drive and other such welfare activities can be sued under the CPA.

STRUCTURE OF CONSUMER FORUMS/COMMISSIONS AND THEIR JURISDICTIONS

	Supreme Court (Final Appeal) ↓	
Appellate Authority over State Commission Revisional Jurisdiction	**National Commission** ↓	Original Jurisdiction Over ₹ 20,00,000
Appellate Authority for District Forum	**State Commission** ↓	Original Jurisdiction over ₹ 5,00,000 up to ₹ 20,00,000
Suo moto Revision	**District Forum**	Original Jurisdiction up to ₹ 5,00,000

The maximum time limit for a claim to be filed under CPA is 2 years from the date of occurrence of the cause of action. There are no court fees to be paid to file a complaint in a Consumer Forum/Commission. Further, a complainant/opposite party can present his case on his own without the help of a lawyer.

As per the Consumer Protection Rules, 1987, a complaint filed in the Consumer Forum/Commission shall be adjudicated, within a period of 90 days from the date of notice by opposite party and within 150 days if it requires analysis or testing of commodities.

THE LEGAL AVENUES (OTHER THAN CPA) AVAILABLE TO AGGRIEVED PATIENTS TO SUE AGAINST HEALTH PROFESSIONALS

1. Medical Council of India and Dental Council of India.
2. Civil Courts.
3. MRTP (Monopolies and Restrictive Trade Practices Commission)
4. Public Interest Litigation.
5. Sections of Indian Penal Code, 1860.
6. Consumer Protection Act, 1986.

REGULATION OF THE PRACTICE OF MEDICINE

Indian Medical Council Act, 1956

Regulates the profession of allopathic medicine by constituting Medical Council of India (MCI) and the State Medical Councils.

Authorizes the Medical Council of India (MCI) to recognize the medical qualifications granted by any Authority or Institution of India or other countries.

- Authorize the MCI to maintain a register of medical practitioners to be known as the Indian Medical register, which consists of the entries of all the State Registers of medical practitioners.
- Empowers the State Medical Councils to punish persons who falsely claim to be registered or misuse titles and when medicine is practiced by unregistered persons, with fine or imprisonment or both.
- Authorizes the MCI to prescribe standards of professional conduct and etiquette or Code of Ethics for medical practitioners. The violations of these standards constitute *infamous conduct (professional misconduct).*

An aggrieved patient can complain to the State Medical Councils about a registered medical practitioner about an alleged wrong committed by him. The Council initiates proper hearing where the concerned doctor is given adequate opportunities to represent his side. If it arrives at the conclusion that the doctor has indeed committed an act, which involves an abuse of professional position that might reasonably by regarded as disgraceful or dishonourable by professional men of good repute and competence, the doctor is either given a warning notice or temporarily or permanently debars him for practicing medicine. The Council does not have any statutory powers to award any compensation to the aggrieved patient or legal heirs. The Indian Medical Council Act, 1956 also provides certain privileges to all the registered medical practitioners.

RIGHTS AND PRIVILEGES OF REGISTERED MEDICAL PRACTITIONERS CONFERRED BY THE INDIAN MEDICAL COUNCIL ACT, 1956

- Right to choose a patient
- Right to add title, descriptions of the academic qualifications to the name
- Right to practice medicine
- Right to dispense medicines
- Right to possess and supply dangerous drugs to the patients

- Right to recovery of fees
- Right for appointment to public and local hospitals
- Right to issue medical certificates
- Right to give evidence as an expert in a court of law.

INDIAN PENAL CODE AND MEDICAL NEGLIGENCE

Indian Penal Code, 1860 sections 52, 80, 81, 83, 88, 90, 91, 92 304-A, 337 and 338 contain the law of medical malpraxis in India.

A physician can be charged with criminal negligence when a patient dies from the effects of anesthesia during an operation or other kind of treatment, if it can be proved that the death was the result if malicious intention, or gross negligence. Before the administration of anesthesia or performance of an operation, the medical man is expected to follow the accepted precautions.

In such cases, the physician should be able to prove that she/he used reasonable and ordinary care in the treatment of his patient to the best of his judgment. She/he is, however, not liable for an error judgment. The law expects a duly qualified physician to use that degree of skill and care which an average man of his qualifications ought to have, and does not expect him to bring the highest possible degree of skill in the treatment of his patients, or to be able to guarantee cures.

It has long been recognized that criminal liability of a physician may result from a high degree of negligent conduct. What the law calls criminal negligence is largely a matter of degree; it is incapable of a precise definition. To prove whether or not it exists is like chasing a mirage. It requires that any of the following to be established in a case of criminal medical negligence.

"Gross lack of competency or gross inattention, or wanton indifferences to the patient's safety, which may arise from gross ignorance of the science of medicine and surgery or through gross negligence, either in the application and selection of remedies, lack of proper skill in the use of instruments and failure to give proper attention to the patient." (Hampton v State [38]; State v Lester).

In RV Bateman (1925), Dr Bateman was prosecuted for manslaughter and the charges of negligence made against him were:

i. Causing the internal ruptures in performing the operations of 'version'.
ii. Removing part of the uterus along with the placenta.
iii. Delay in sending the patient to the infirmary.

The trial court convicted him. But the Court of Appeal held: " ... in order to establish criminal liability, the facts must be such that, .. the negligence of the accused went beyond a mere matter of compensation between subjects and should such disregard for the life and safety of others as to amount to a crime against the State and conduct punishment."

When a FIR (First Information Report) is filed against a doctor for the death of a patient who was under his treatment, under this Indian Penal Code Section 304-A the doctor can be arrested. A doctor charged under this section can obtain bail and if proved guilty, the doctor can be punished with a maximum of two years imprisonment or fine or both. But, if the patient is alive, the doctor is charged under the Indian Penal Code Section 337 and 338.

The Indian Courts have been very careful not to hold qualified physicians criminally (instances of quacks for criminal negligence are there) liable for patients' deaths that are the result of a mere mistake of judgment in the selection and application of remedies and when the death resulted merely from an error of judgment or an inadvertent death.

DO'S AND DON'TS FOR DOCTORS

DO'S FOR DOCTORS

- Mention your qualifications/training/experience/designation on the prescription. Qualifications mean recognized degrees/diplomas as regulated by the Indian Medical Degrees Act, 1916 as amended from time to time. Mention of scholarships/membership/awards which are no qualifications should be avoided
- Always mention date and time of the consultation
- Mention age and sex of the patient. In a pediatric prescription weight of the patient must also be mentioned
- Always check with hand on the part that the patient/attendant says is painful. Use stethoscope to check, even if for cosmetic reasons
- Listen attentively. Look carefully. Ask questions intelligently
- If, after completing the examination, the patient/attendant feels that something has been left out or wants something to be examined, oblige him
- Always face the patient. Do not stare. Some patients tolerate very little eye contact. Learn to observe out of the corner of our eyes
- In case you have been distracted/inattentive during the history taking, ask the patient/attendant to start all over again. She/he will never mind it. As far as possible consultations should not be interrupted for non-urgent calls

- Ask the patient to come back for review the next day, in case She/he was examined hurriedly or if you are not sure about the diagnosis/treatment
- Mention "diagnosis under review" until the diagnosis is finally settled
- In complicated cases, record precisely the history of illness and substantial physical findings about the patient on your prescription
- If the patient/attendants are erring on any count (history not reliable, refusing investigations, refusing admission) make a note of it or seek written refusal preferably in local language with proper witness
- Mention the condition of patient in specific/objective terms. Avoid vague/nonspecific terminology
- Record history of drug allergy
- Write names of drugs clearly. Use correct dosages (by revising knowledge periodically) and mention clearly method and interval of administration. Here one must use local or sign language. Do not forget writing precautions like Ast/pc/ac/locally/with milk/hs, etc. in local language
- If a drug is a poison (e.g. certain local applications), warn in writing
- Mention additional precautions e.g. food, rest, avoidance of certain drugs, allergens, alcohol, smoking, etc. if indicated
- Give instruction to the patient in comprehensible terms, making sure that the patient understands both the instruction and the importance of strictly adhering to them. For example while prescribing to potent anti-inflammatory drug, warn that if he experience any stomach trouble he should stop taking the drug and consult a doctor immediately
- Mention likely side effects, and action to be taken if they occur
- Remember to advise in writing pathological tests/radiological tests at specified intervals for certain drugs which require such monitoring if such drugs are prescribed. Some examples are: sodium valporate, carbamezapine, gold salts, methotrexate and other immuno-suppressives, chloramphemicol, etc.
- Always advise the patient not to stop taking a drug suddenly which is required to be tapered before it is stopped. Remember major drug interactions
- Specifically mention review, SOS/or follow-up schedule
- Mention if patient/attendant are/is under effect of alcohol/drugs
- In case a particular drug/equipment is not available, make a note
- Prescribe with caution during pregnancy/lactation
- Adjust doses in case of a child/elderly patient and in renal or hepatic disorders

- In case of chronic ailments, mention treatment to be taken immediately in case of an emergency. For example, a patient on antiepileptic treatment should be advised to take an injection of diazepam when convulsions occur. In case of any deviation from standard care, mention reasons
- Mention whether prognosis explained. If necessary take a signature of patient/attendant, after explaining the prognosis in written local language. Mention where the patient should contact in case of your nonavailability/ emergency
- If you are not sure what disease a patient has after a through work-up, get a consultation. Develop a lost of physicians you trust and respect in each of the specialties. Nurture your relationship with them, and consult them about difficult cases
- Whenever referring a patient, provide him with a referring note. In case of emergency/serious illness, ring up the concerned doctor in the patient's presence. Show your concern. Always keep with you and refer the latest edition of the standard text book of your branch of medicine. Always subscribe to at least one standard journal and participate in at least updates/ conferences every year
- Update your knowledge and skill from time to time. If a doctor does not keep pace with recent advances, the quality of care suffers and does not measure upto the standards of reasonable care and skill. Many doctors tend to deteriorate in their knowledge, skills and attitude, over a period to time. Not only do they not make any attempt to update themselves but they slip downwards (doctors may become incompetent due to other causes: age, mental illness, addiction to alcohol or drug abuse)
- Update not only your own knowledge and skill, but also that of your staff. Update the facilities and equipment according to prevailing current standards in your area
- Preferably employ qualified assistants. If not available, impart proper training and skill at your or some appropriate centre and obtain a certificate for the same
- Medication to relieve pain especially in postoperative and cancer cases must be carried our carefully
- Always obtain a legally valid consent before undertaking surgical/ diagnostic procedure. Learn the difference between "informed persuasion" and "informed consent". The first is legally wrong, through at times it may be medically correct (For details on consent, see under "Preventive Steps Against Litigation" in "Medical Profession and Consumer Protection Act", 1994 edn.). In case of MTP/sterilization, always follow the guidelines

issued by the Government of India in Medical Profession and Consumer Protection Act, 1994 edn.)

- While administering an injection/vaccination always check:
  1. Name of the injection (a wrong injection may be given by mistake or oversight).
  2. Expiry date.
  3. Reconfirm the route of administration.
  4. If it is to be diluted, check the dilution factor (1:2, 1:4, etc.).
  5. Rate of administration (fast, slow, in drip, etc.).
  6 Site of infection, e.g. antero-lateral, thigh, if age 1 year, gluteal region, deltoid, etc.
  7. That a disposable syringe and needle are used. If that is not possible, use syringe and needle after proper sterilization.
  8. In case the patient is agitated/not cooperating, restrain him properly with 1 or 2 assistants or wait until he calms down. It is not unusual for a broken needle leaking to a claim for compensation.
  9. Confirm that it has been kept at the required temperature.
  10 If required to be reconstituted, check the diluent and whether it has got to be cooled before using.
  11. Routinely advise X-rays in injury to bones and joints and related diseases of bones/joints.
  12. Always rule out pregnancy before subjecting the uterus to X-ray. Always read reports carefully and interpret the results of tests/X-rays properly and make a note of it.
  13. In all instances of "swab cases" and "instrument cases", the surgeon in charge has been directly or vicariously held liable for negligence. The surgeon in charge must therefore personally ensure that such mishaps do not occur. The period for the responsibility of the surgeon extends to and includes the postoperative care. He must therefore ensure proper postoperative care to the patient.
  14. Always seek proper legal and medical advice before filing reply to the complainant referred to you from a consumer court.

DON'TS FOR DOCTORS

- Do not prescribe without examining the patient, even if he is a close friend or relative (Telephone advice is an exception)
- Never examine a female patient without presence of female nurse/ attendant, especially during genital and breast examinations

- Do not insist on the patient to tell the history of illness or be examined in presence of others. He has right to privacy and confidentiality
- Do not permit considerations of religion, nationality, race, party, politics or social standing to intervene between you and your patient
- It may not be reasonable for a doctor to assume what the patient is saying is truthful where what the patient/attendant says is clearly contradicted by the symptoms
- Do not smoke while examining a patient
- Do not examine a patient when you are sick, exhausted, or under influence of alcohol or any intoxicated substance
- Do not be overconfident. Do not look overconfident
- Do not prescribe a drug or indulge in a procedure of you cannot justify its indication
- Do not prescribe a drug or indulge in a procedure of you cannot justify its indication
- Do not prescribe/administer a drug which is banned, for example Analgin
- Do not over-prescribe/administer: too much of the drug, too large a dose, for too long
- Do not under-prescribe: not prescribing the needed drug, dose is too small, length of treatment is too short
- Do not prescribe multiple drugs. Such prescription may be due to inability to form a correct diagnosis or other causes. Possibilities of drug interactions increase with polypharmacy
- Do not write instructions on a separate slip. Do not allow substitutions
- Do not adopt experimental method in treatment. If there is some rationale do it only after informed consent
- Do not do anything beyond your level of competence. Competence is defined by your qualification, training and experience
- Do not give a drug parenterally if it can be given orally. There may be some exceptions
- When you are not sure what and why to do. Consult your senior/ specialist/ colleague
- Do not refuse if the patient/attendants want to leave against medical advice. It is their right. Document this properly
- Never avoid a call for help from a nurse on duty at night. In all probability a genuine emergency may be there
- Never order an investigation unless the result is likely to help you direct the treatment or make a difference in what you tell a patient

- Do not allow modern diagnostics tests to substitute clinical judgment. At best, they can only supplement. Always analyze the cost-benefit ratio before rushing to get these tests done. In case a particular test has had high false positive or false-negative results, explain this to the patient before getting it done
- Never label any condition as "functional" until you are as certain as possible of the accuracy
- Do not withhold information, however harsh and difficult, in seriously/ terminally ill patients. It must be conveyed with compassion and gradually, if time permits. The doctors and especially their assistants must train themselves in the art of sensitive communication. It would be wise to take into confidence the family members, close relatives and friends, this would often make the acceptance easier and quicker
- Do not leave at the moment of death. There is a tendency especially on the part of senior doctors to go away at this time when his presence and experience are most needed
- Do not hesitate to extend your condolences and sympathies to the bereaved persons
- Do not forget to provide genetic counseling to couples and parents with known family history/ children having genetic abnormalities, for examples: Thalassemia, Hemophilia, etc
- Do not issue death certificates unless you have yourself verified it
- Do not divulge secrets you come to know during discharge of your professional duties. There are five exceptions to this general principle;
  1. If the patient gives consent
  2. When it is undesirable on medical grounds to seek a patient's consent
  3. The information is required by due legal process
  4. For the purposes of medical research, after obtaining permission from competent authority.
- Do not deny medical care to a patient with HIV infection/AIDS. Observe all necessary precautions.
- Do not inform that the person is infected with HIV unless confirmatory test results are received. Do not give untrue, misleading or improper reports, documents, etc.
- Do not refuse the patient's right to examine and receive an explanation about your bill regardless of the source of payment; whether or not it is reimbursed by the government or by his employer/insurance company.
- Do not refuse the patient's right to know about the hospital rules and regulations.

- Never talk loose of your colleagues, despite intense professional rivalry. Never criticize others in profession. The patient/attendants may incite you to say/do something. They may seek your comments on the other doctor's treatment. There is always a polite way to set aside their comments and queries. Remember if you have seen the case from the start you would have done the same. If your colleague has made an error of judgment regarding diagnosis or treatment, you never know under what circumstances this has happened.

PREVENTIVE MEASURES (HOW TO AVOID LITIGATION)

GENERAL GUIDELINES FOR LEGAL DEFENSE

Not defending yourself and hospital is negligence. We should always make all possible points in defense in first instance of making a reply to the complainant. Subsequent points during hearing of the case are liable to be rejected.

TECHNICAL DEFENSES AND FACTUAL DEFENSES

Technical Defenses

1. The medical service rendered was free of charge (now, this is applicable in certain situations only).
2. Concurrent adjudication in another court.
3. The court does not have pecuniary/territorial jurisdiction.
4. Complaint is time-barred.
5. Complicate issues involved, required recording of evidence of experts, hence case should relegated to a civil court. Such a plea must be taken at the beginning of the trial.
6. The complaints frivolous and vexations and liable to be dismissed under Section 26 of the Act.
7. Inform the insurance company in writing with a copy of the complaint in case of any insurance policy takes for professional indemnity.

Factual Defenses

1. Mention qualifications, training, experience, expertise etc.of professionals Support with relevant documents.
2. Mention hospitals infrastructure facilities, special facilities, back-up support with documents.
3. If Complainant has suppressed material facts before the court of law i.e previous illness, treatment, etc.

4. Inconsistence between notices sent directly or through consumer groups and the complaint made in the court.
5. Written evidence of consent of the patient/relative/attendant to assumption of inherent and special risks in the treatment.
6. Circumstances of the case; viz. There was emergency, lack of facilities (e.g. rural area) no one to give history of patient's illness, etc.
7. Burden of proof of: (i) duty of care (ii) breach of that duty (iii) causation (iv) damage, etc. is on the complainant.
8. Reasonable knowledge, skill and care exercised (Rely/quote standard text books with attested photocopies).
9. Consolation/treatment by patient from other doctor/other systems of medicine simultaneously.
10. Many other reasons/more than one reason/for occurrence of damage.
11. Contributory negligence.

CHAPTER 21

Personnel Management

One of the important functions of the personnel department is manpower planning.

Manpower planning may be defined as a technique for the procurement, development, allocation and utilization of human resources in an organization.

It is also described as the manpower management, which means it is basically concerned with engaging the right type of personnel for the right job at the right time. This can be done by studying the following forecasts.

1. Economic forecast
2. Hospitals expansion forecast
3. Employees market forecast
4. Anticipating from past records

a. Resignations
b. Dismissals
c. Retirements/retrenchments.

FUNCTIONS

Manpower planning covers the total activity of the personnel functions such as recruitment, selection, training, career development and staff appraisal.

Manpower planning involves the following steps:

a. Scrutiny of the present personnel strength
b. Anticipation of manpower needs
c. Investigation of the turnover of personnel
d. Planning job requirements and job description.

Some of the important factors which result in employee turnover are:

1. Low salary
2. Better prospects in other hospitals
3. Poor working conditions
4. Transport problems
5. Housing problem
6. In case of female employees—marriage and pregnancy
7. Health grounds
8. Family problems
9. Seeking higher education
10. Ill treatment by the superiors
11. Unfriendly relationship with colleagues
12. Going back to ones native place and
13. Job opportunity in foreign countries.

Hence, the management should have an exit interview with all the employees at the time of leaving organization. It helps the management to understand reason for employee turnover and thereby to take measures to prevent such happening in future wherever possible. It also helps in reducing employee turnover and builds the morale of employees working in the hospital.

HUMAN RESOURCE MANAGEMENT

The requirement for human resources should be analyzed before recruiting and selecting manpower for the hospital. The number of employees required for each category of employees for all the departments is decided based on:

a. The size of the hospital
b. The locality of hospital
c. Type of hospital
d. Degree of care that is provided
e. Type of equipments
f. Type of building structures (horizontal/vertical)
g. Size of campus, etc.

While calculating the number of employees required, the number of female staff should be taken into account for the purpose of calculating maternity leave, general leave vacancy and also the percentage of habitual absenteeism.

The general ratio of employees per bed is 1:2 or 1:3 (Here employee means all the persons working in hospital whether medical, para medical, service, maintenance, administration, accounts, staff, etc.)

DIFFERENCE BETWEEN HUMAN RESOURCE MANAGEMENT AND PERSONNEL MANAGEMENT

Human resource management deals with manpower planning, recruitment, selection, orientation, training, performance appraisal, promotions, transfers and separations.

Personnel management deals with the function of HR manager. It also deals with salary administration, working conditions, safety, welfare, health services, communication, counseling, collective bargaining, disciplinary actions and personnel audit.

The human resource deals only with bright side of the personal activities and personnel management deals with the bright as well as dark side of the personnel activities of an organization.

Human resource management is a narrow term whereas personnel management is a wider term.

INDUCTION PROGRAMS

In any organization, induction program is one of the important functions of the personnel department.

In hospitals, induction program is very important and essential for smooth functioning of the hospital.

INDUCTION

The process of induction is carried out to help a new employee to fit smoothly into the functioning of the hospital. She/he is introduced to the existing employees so that she/he may develop a sense of belonging. This induction sequence aim at helping the new employee visualize her/his place in the overall hospital functioning.

In induction programs an employee is introduced to the following:

a. Introduction to a brief history of the hospital.
b. Creating awareness about its aim and objectives.
c. The terms and conditions of the appointment letter.
d. Personnel policy.
e. The scope of services available in the hospital.
f. The personnel benefits available to the employee.
g. The attitude expected from the employee with regard to patients and visitors.
h. Promotion policy.
i. Names of key officials.

j. His/her position in the hierarchy
k. Fire safety precaution and safety regulations
l. Introducing the costaff working in the department where she/he is posted and
m. Orientation about the hospital departments and layout of the hospital.

It has been observed in many hospitals the consultants and other staff move in the corridors and in the same premises of the hospital but they many not know each other. Sometimes, the consultants refer patients to other specialists but when they come across in the corridors or in the wards they do not greet each other as they may not know even such specialist consultant is available in the hospital.

The officer has to introduce herself/himself to the new staff when she/he visits the department (if proper induction is not carried out).

Hence, induction is extremely important in a hospital for co-operation, and coordination among the staff and also for smooth functioning of the hospital.

It is the duty of the personnel manager to conduct induction programme for the new staff as per the schedule,

If the hospital authorities take note of the following points, they can certainly get the best out of their employees.

1. The physical surroundings in which employees do their jobs must be as pleasant and comfortable.
2. Adequate welfare services such as staff quarters, transport, canteen, counseling, etc. should be provided.
3. The number of working hours should be not more than 48 hours in a week. This helps in getting efficient work and avoids fatigue in the work.
4. Security of employment in all respects must be provided by the hospital authorities.
5. The employee safety and their health should be ensured.

NURSES AND DOCTORS TO BED RATIO

The number of nurses required depends on the number of wards, number of beds in each ward, number of ICU beds, CCU beds, number of operation theaters, types of beds (general, single, room, etc). The number of nurses and paramedical staff required for a ward consisting of 10–12 beds is given in the table below:

WARDS

	General shift	Morning shift	Evening shift	Night relievers	Total
Ward in-charge nursing officer	1	—	—	—	1
Staff nurse	2	2	1	1	6
Paramedical ANM/nurses	1	1	1		3
Ward boy/aya	2	2	1	1	6
MNA	1	—	—	—	1

For every six employees of the same category, one reliever is to be provided. Wherever the number is less than 6, one reliever is posted for 2 wards, nursing superintendent will have separate staff as relievers in each category like nurses, ANMs, 'ayahs', 'boys'. They are posted to the wards wherever there is a need.

ICU/emergency ward with 7 ventilated patients and 4 nonventilated patients.

	GS	MS	ES	NS	R	Total
Ward Incharge	1					1
Batch Incharge		1	1	1		3
Nurses		9	9	9	5	32
Ayah/ward boy		3	3	2	1	9

One nurse is posted for every patient with ventilator in ICU and one nurse for two patients without ventilator should be posted.

Generally one nursing station is be provided for one ward consisting of 12 beds and for more than 12, it would be difficult to monitor patients and give best services to the patients by nurses and other paramedical staff. If the beds are more than 12 and less than 20, one more sub-station should be provided which will work under the control of one ward In-charge.

Number of staff required for the ward also depends upon the type of ward. If the ward is a general ward where the beds are arranged one by one in a big hall with common toilets, the staff requirement is less.

If the ward is with single rooms with attached bathrooms and toilets the staff requirement is more.

In the ward where more equipments are used, the staff requirement is more than the single room ward.

DOCTORS TO BED RATIO

Here doctor means resident medical officer or duty medical officer. Generally for every 10–12 beds one medical officer is posted to look after the patients admitted in that particular ward. If a doctor has to look after more than 10–12 patients, he will not be able to do full justice to the patients. But this ratio is not to be applicable for high risk wards like ICU, casualty, Isolation ward, etc. The RMO should be posted in the wards round the clock. In case of shortage of doctors, at least RMOs should be available between 8 am to 8 pm in the ward. In case of night emergencies, ward in-charge can call the doctors in ICU for assessment and patient can be shifted to the ICU/emergency ward.

DUTIES AND RESPONSIBILITIES OF PERSONNEL MANAGER

1. Anticipating and providing data for future openings.
2. Seeking and attracting qualified applicants to fill the vacancies.
3. Determining the organizational structure and manpower needs to effectively meet the organizational objectives.
4. Analyzing the applicants qualifications for determining their suitability.
5. Officially assigning each employee an appropriate position which clearly defines his/her responsibilities.
6. Ensuring that new recruits are provided with appropriate training and information to enable them to perform their duties effectively and thereby using their potential to the maximum.
7. Providing training for the individual employee's development.
8. Arranging programs as per the requirements of developing existing personnel.
9. Providing facilities for job satisfaction and making the workplace more attractive.
10. Providing the needed exchange of information throughout the organization.
11. Building rapport with the officially-recognized and legally established employees' organizations in the best interests of both the organization and its employees.
12. Developing effective work regulations and harmonious work relationships.

13. Objectively apprising each employees performance in relation to the duties and the responsibilities assigned.
14. Helping employees in solving their personal problems.
15. Developing facilities and procedures for the prevention of on-the-job accidents.
16. Preventing diseases and physical ailments and at the same time caring for diseases, ailments and injuries suffered by employees on the job.
17. Providing precautionary measures for safeguarding the organization and its property from fire, theft, etc.
18. Developing/improving employees attitudes and conditions of work.
19. Conducting personnel audit.

DUTIES OF HUMAN RESOURCE MANAGER

The HR manager manages the day-to-day operations of the human resources office. The HR generalist manages the administration of the human resources policies, procedures and programes. The HR manager carries out the responsibilities in the following functional areas: departmental development, human resource information systems (HRIS), employee relations, training and development, benefits compensation, organizational development/ employment.

The HR manager is responsible for all or part of these areas:

1. Recruiting and staffing logistics.
2. Organizational and space planning.
3. Performance management and improvement systems.
4. Organization development.
5. Employment and compliance to regulatory concerns and reporting.
6. Employee orientation, development and training.
7. Policy development and documentation.
8. Employee relations.
9. Hospitals wide committee facilitation.
10. Hospital employee communication.
11. Compensation and benefits administration.
12. Employee safety, welfare, wellness and health.
13. Employee services and counseling.

The manager originates and leads human resources practices and objectives that provide an employee-oriented, high performance culture that emphasizes empowerment, quality, productivity and standards, goal attainment and the recruitment and ongoing development of a superior workforce.

He coordinates implementation of services, policies, and programs through human resources staff; reports to the human resources director, and assists and advises hospital managers about human resources issues.

Primary objectives of the HR portfolio are:

- Safety of the workforce
- Development of a superior workforce
- Development of the human resource department
- Development of an employee oriented hospital culture that emphasizes quality, continuous improvement, and high performance
- Personal ongoing development.

DISCIPLINE AND DISCIPLINARY ACTION

INTRODUCTION

Discipline means orderliness. It is the primary responsibility of the management to maintain discipline in an organisation. In doing so, it must make its standards known to its employees. If employees do not know what standards the management expects from them, their conduct is likely to be misdirected. The management should maintain discipline by applying standards in a consistent, fair and flexible manner.

As orderly behavior is essential for attaining the organization's objectives, all employees must be disciplined. Discipline should be administered by the management without favoritism and partiality. Successful executives direct discipline against an act of misconduct and not against any person.

COMPLAINT PROCEDURE

All complaints arising out of employment, including those relating to unfair treatment or wrongful exacting of money on the part of the management, should preferably be referred to the head of the department in which the employee works. In the event that the employee is not satisfied with the department head's decision or if the latter so wishes, the complaint should be referred to the chief executive of the hospital. The chief executive may, at her/his discretion, appoint an officer or a committee to investigate the complaint; or after a formal enquiry by the personnel officer, communicate her/his decision to the employee through the head of department.

If a superior has any complaint against her/his subordinate for not carrying out the instructions, or if a patient has a complaint against any employee of the hospital, the management must obtain the complaint in writing and should avoid taking action on an oral complaint. This sort of complaint should always be addressed to the chief executive of the hospital who has hiring and firing authority.

PRELIMINARY ENQUIRY

In cases of misconduct, before the chief executive decides to issue a formal charge-sheet and holds a regular enquiry, She/he should try to determine whether there is a prima facie case against the accused employee by ordering a preliminary enquiry. If it is found that the allegation against her/him is of a minor nature not warranting disciplinary action, she/he should be let off with a warning. But if the misconduct appears to be of grave nature, a regular enquiry should be initiated on the basis of the evidence available at the preliminary enquiry.

Holding of a preliminary enquiry is always desirable because holding a regular enquiry is a serious matter which can cause unrest or have other undesirable effects. But a preliminary enquiry has its limitations. No employee can be punished on the findings of a preliminary enquiry. An employee can be exonerated or punished only after of a regular enquiry.

DISCIPLINARY ACTION

Disciplinary action is generally confined to the punishment of the erring employee to prevent his undesirable behavior in future. Though the majority of employees confirm to orders, policies, and rules and regulations, the erring minority does require disciplinary action.

PROCEDURE FOR DISCIPLINARY ACTION

The management starts the procedure of disciplinary action against an employee by issuing a charge-sheet. It gives an opportunity to an employee to explain his conduct. Therefore, it is sometimes called a 'show cause notice'.

If the charges are of a very serious nature, the employee should be suspended as well, so that he may not tamper with the records and mislead witnesses.

Thus, a domestic enquiry first requires the framing of the charges with details of the offence in the form of a charge-sheet requiring the employee to show cause as to why appropriate action should not be taken against him. After the charge-sheeted employee has given his written explanation, it should be examined. In case the explanation given by the employee is not satisfactory, an enquiry letter should be issued, giving him reasonable time (minimum 72 hours) to prepare his case and to arrange his witnesses, if any.

A person who conducts an enquiry is called an enquiry officer. He should be impartial and qualified to act in that capacity. An enquiry officer can be disqualified on any of the following grounds:

1. If he is personally involved in the concerned incident which is being enquired into.
2. If he has personal knowledge of the incident.
3. If he has collected evidence on behalf of the management for the very enquiry being conducted by him.

When the enquiry officer commences enquiry, she/he should mark the presence of the management's representative and the charge—sheeted employee and his representative, if any. He should then read out the charges as contained in the charge-sheet. After that he should ask the charge-sheeted employee whether he confesses to or denies the charges. If the charge-sheeted employee confesses to the charges, the enquiry officer should record his statement obtain the signatures of the charge-sheeted employee and the management's representative, and submit his report to the chief executive of the hospital.

If the charge-sheeted employee denies the charges, the enquiry officer should direct the management's representative to present the case of the management. At this stage, the management's representative should file documents and examine all witnesses of the management, one by one to prove the charges. The enquiry officer should allow the charged-sheeted employee to cross examine every witness of the management after recording the statement of each witness.

Once the management's representative has completed the presentation of the case on behalf of the management by filing documents and presenting all witnesses one by one, the enquiry officer should call upon the charge-sheeted employee to present his defence by filing documents, if any, by giving his own statement and producing his witnesses. After recording the Statement of every witness produced by the charge-sheeted employee, he should ask the management's representative to cross-examine them.

On completion of the examination, cross-examination, etc. of the witnesses of both sides, the enquiry officer hears argument and writes an enquiry report and submit it alongwith the enquiry proceedings to the chief executive of the institution. In his report, he concludes whether the charges are proved or disproved. The decision about the enquiry or penalty rests with the chief executive.

The personnel officer must give due attention to the likely repercussions on discipline and general relationships in the organization while advising management whether to proceed or not with a disciplinary case. Even where there is solid proof against an employee, it should be considered whether an enquiry is advisable or whether some other line of action may prove more effective in improving discipline for the future; such as consultation with the trade union or the works committee in the hope that social pressure may be brought upon the delinquent employee to apologize and not to repeat the misconduct. Departmental enquiry has now become so complicated that it may or may not be upheld by the labour courts. If disciplinary action is not taken, other employees are likely to make the allegation that the guilty employee is a favourite of the management or that the management is incapable of taking any action against him. However, before taking any disciplinary action it is advisable to properly weigh the gravity of the misconduct and the result which disciplinary action taken against an employee is likely to have on the morale of the employees. It would be better if social pressure is generated, so that the delinquent employee either leaves the institution or apologizes in writing.

FORMS OF PUNISHMENT

Generally, the forms of punishment are as laid down in the certified standing orders of the establishment. In the absence of the certified standing otders, the model standing orders prescribed by the state government under the provision of 'The Industrial Employment (Standing Orders) Act, 1946' shall form the basis for pronouncing the punishment.

The forms of punishment are as follows:

Warning: This is a bad remark in the personnel file of an employee and is a sort of stigma in his service record.

Fine: In certain cases, an employee is fined for his misconduct. Fine should be imposed in the manner and to the extent laid down in the Payment of Wages Act, 1936. The maximum fine permitted tobe deducted according to the Payment of Wages Act, 1936, is 3 paise in a rupee from the employee's salary.

Suspension: An employee may be suspended pending enquiry. He could also be suspended as a punishment. The certified standing orders of every establishment should specifically prescribe the number of days for which such punishment can be imposed.

Termination: Similarly, there can be a provision in the personnel policies for termination of service of an employee (not applicable to supervisory and managerial staff) by giving one month's notice or one month's pay in lieu thereof.

Grounds of dismissal: There are certain acts of misconduct which warrant dismissal. Some of them are (a) willful insubordination or disobedience (b) theft, fraud or dishonesty in connection with the employer's business or property (c) willful damage or loss of employer's goods or property (d) taking or giving bribes (e) habitual unauthorized absence or late attendance (f) habitual breach of any law (g) riotous or disorderly behavior during working hours or any act subversive of discipline (h) striking work or inciting others to strike work.

Whenever an employee commits any of the aforesaid acts of misconduct, he should be charge-sheeted, an enquiry to be held and a dismissal order be passed if the charge is proved.

Some guiding principles in dismissal cases

No employer should dismiss an employee during the pendency of his proceedings in any other matter before a conciliation officer, labour court or industrial tribunal without seeking express permission of the concerned court under Section 33 (1) of the Industrial Disputes Act, 1947.

During the pendency of any notice of general demands before a conciliation officer, labor court or industrial tribunal, an employer can dismiss an employee but should take approval of the concerned court, under section 33(2) of the Industrial Disputes Act, 1947.

Grounds of discharge: Both discharge and dismissal result in the termination of service of an employee, but there is a substantial difference between the two. Discharge is nothing more than a termination of services of an employee with full rights such as provident fund, gratuity, service compensation at the rate of 15 days' salary for every completed year of service under Section 25 (f) of the Industrial Disputes Act, 1947, and one month's notice pay. Thus discharge of an employee is also known as discharge simpliciter.

Dismissal, on the other hand, is termination of the services of an employee by way of punishment which deprives him of a number of benefits. As a matter of fact, both kinds of termination of service are disciplinary actions for the misconduct of an employee, but dismissal is the most severe punishment which should be imposed upon an employee only in extreme circumstances.

In awarding punishment under the personnel policies, the chief executive should take into account the gravity of misconduct, the previous record, if any, of the employee and any other extenuating circumstances that may exist. The reasons for the termination of service may be grave, but depending on the consequences of the misconduct and the motive behind it, the management at their discretion may order discharge instead of dismissal.

The services of an employee may be terminated in cases of habitual negligence of work, undue extension of leave, inefficiency, suspected loyalty, etc.

Grounds of warning: For most cases, an oral warning is sufficient to achieve the desired result. The supervisor must know his subordinate, and how to give a warning. If the misconduct is more serious, the reprimand may be put in writing. Since a written warning is more permanent than an oral one, it is considered a severe penalty. For such offences as tardiness, leaving the workplace without permission and smoking in the wards, written warning can be given. If an employee has been consistently sincere throughout his service, he may be let off with a warning, even for a serious misconduct. He may also be let off with a warning if he confesses the charges and tenders an unconditional apology.

CONCLUSION

After the disciplinary action, the supervisor should assume a normal attitude towards the employee treating the chapter as closed. If the supervisor continues to regard the employee with suspicion, the employee will feel uneasy while working; distrust between the supervisor and employee should be avoided at all costs.

One thing to remember while taking disciplinary action is that the procedure for disciplinary action should be based on principles of natural justice: an opportunity must be given to the employee to show cause; no decision should be taken by someone who is biased; no decision impairing any person's rights should be based on inaccurate facts; and the employee is entitled to know the reason for any decision.

However, the attitude of the supervisor should be one of counseling and understanding rather than 'police and punish'. Her/his goal should be to effect a change for greater consistency with the organization's requirements. She/he should try to achieve this through counseling. When he fails to bring about the desired change in an employee, She/he should adopt disciplinary procedure as a last resort.

CHAPTER 22

Finance Management

Management of finance in any organization deals with costing, budgeting, accounting with the final object of giving net profit to the organization. In hospitals, finance department plays major role in monitoring and controlling hospital funds. In a financially unsound organization growth is not possible.

The service organizations which run on public funds or donations are exempted from this law. Some organizations which are service oriented, are run on sponsors or donations from philanthropists. General administration, medical administration, finance management and personnel management are some of the important areas in hospital administration. The administrators of the hospitals are qualified and specialized in hospital administration. Medical administrators like medical superintendents, nursing superintendents, and doctors, etc. are specialists in the field of medicine. So far no specialized courses for hospital finance management and hospital personnel management are offered in India. As it is already mentioned at the beginning of this chapter, the two fields of management finance and personnel are common to all the organizations except in the area of inputs and expectations. Hospital finance and personnel department are usually managed by virtue of experience by the person appointed by the board members.

DIFFERENCES BETWEEN HOSPITAL MANAGEMENT AND THE MANAGEMENT OF OTHER ORGANIZATION

1. Revenue is generated to the hospital from the inpatients, the outpatients' treatment and other supportive services.

   Revenue is generated in other profit making bodies from the sale of products or the sale of services.

2. The Services are restricted to a particular place city or customers in the area.
   The sale of products is in a particular region or throughout the country.
3. Revenue depends on the quality of services provided to the patients. Revenue depends on the quality of products provided to the customers.
4. Hospitals deal with human lives, whereas industries are deal with men and materials.
5. Raw materials are essential to get the final product in an industry. drugs and professional services are required to treat the illness of the patient.

SOURCES OF INCOME IN THE HOSPITALS

The sources of income in the hospitals are from:

1. Inpatient treatment which includes:
   - Bed charges
   - Nursing/service
   - Investigation
   - Oxygen
   - Monitor, ventilator, pulse oxymeters
   - Procedures
   - Diet
   - Medicines from the pharmacy
   - Operation theater charges
   - Drugs used in OT
   - Professional charges
   - Physiotherapy charges
   - Blood bank charges
   - Cost of implants (if any)
   - Instrument charges
   - Package charges (if any)
   - Other.
2. Outpatient charges which include:
   - Registration
   - Procedures
   - Dressing
   - Professional fees
   - Investigation
   - Pharmacy medicines

- Physiotherapy charges, etc.
- Even the charges for the food in the canteen comes in this category.

3. From outside referral patients include:
   - Investigation
   - Physiotherapy charges
   - Blood bank charges
   - Master health checkup
   - Rentals/maintenance charges from doctors or others for facilities provided
   - Income from outsourced departments is also come under this category.

UTILIZATION OF FUNDS

The revenue of the hospital is to be spent/utilized under the following heads of expenditure:

1. Establishment/salaries to the staff
2. Welfare facilities to staff
3. Electricity charges
4. Maintenance charges
5. Transport/vehicle maintenance
6. Oxygen charges
7. Air conditioning charges
8. Insurance for equipment
9. Service charges/AMCs
10. Replacement of spares
11. Housekeeping charges
12. Printing and stationery
13. Professional charges
14. Licenses and taxes
15. Employee's provident fund
16. ESI payment
17. Canteen expenses
18. Audit fees.

In addition to the above expenditure the following capital expenditure is essential in the following areas:

1. Replacement of medical equipments
2. Purchase of new and latest technology equipments
3. Air conditioners

4. Computers
5. Hospital furniture and fixtures, etc.
6. Generators
7. Motors
8. Electrification, etc.
9. Expansion of buildings
10. Modification of buildings
11. Vehicles, ambulences, etc.

One of the areas where a hospital should concentrate more is on sundry debtors who are mostly public sector undertakings, companies, TPA's, insurance companies, etc. They send their employees or card holders to the hospital for their treatment or treatment to their dependants on credit/cashless basis. The companies settle the bills to the hospital as per the terms and conditions mentioned in the MOU. The companies or PSUs, TPA companies, take minimum of 15 days to 30 days for making payments to the hospital. Sometimes, it may even be extended to 45 days as clarification regarding charges is needed.

STATUTORY PAYMENTS

The finance manager should concentrate on monthly/periodical statutory payments to the Government IT Department and other revenue departments. They are:

1. Monthly TDS on staff salaries to be paid to income tax department.
2. Monthly TDS on Professional fees paid to the doctors.
3. Monthly TDS to the contractors.
4. TDS on Service contractors (AMCs).
5. TDS on rentals, if any.
6. Service tax, if applicable on any services.
7. Provident fund.
8. ESI.
9. Corporation tax.
10. Water and sewage charges.
11. Urban land tax, if any.
12. License fees for renewal of various licenses like, drug license, blood bank license, etc.
13. Pollution control board, etc.

DUTIES AND RESPONSIBILITIES OF THE CHIEF FINANCE OFFICER OR THE DIRECTOR—FINANCE AND ACCOUNTS

1. The CFO or director of finance and accounts is the overall in charge of the finance and the accounts of the departments of the hospital.
2. She/he should ensure that all departments functioning under him are working smoothly, economically and efficiently.
3. She/he should be organize and supervise all hospital purchases, coordinate with the respective staff. This may include includes purchase of medical equipment, nonmedical items, stationery.
4. She/he should monitor to the department under his control. She/he must also do surprise checks of stores, accounts, billing and cash counters.
5. She/he should to see that all accounting records are in order and upto date.
6. She/he should prepare an annual budget for the hospital.
7. In stores, he should ensure that all inventory of consumable and non-consumable items including fixed assets are in order. Any theft/loss/damages should investigated by him/her promptly and proper action must be immediately taken.
8. She/he plans and coordinates all the financial transactions of the hospital and undertakes future budgeting.
9. It should be duty of the finance and accounts officer to see that AMC's of various equipments are up-to-date and are in order.
10. She/he should monitor the corporate billing section regarding the credit bills raised on various companies and Insurance companies and the payments received from them.
11. She/he should send reminders to the concerned parties/public sector undertaking or insurance companies for payments in case of huge outstanding amounts.
12. She/he should ensure that the statutory requirements like the periodical Statements/returns like TDS, service tax, sales tax, etc. are submitted to the respective departments without fail along with the payment.
13. She/he should check the cash deposits and cheque deposits in the bank.
14. She/he should monitor the day today expenditure of the hospital.

DUTIES AND RESPONSIBILITIES OF MANAGER/ACCOUNTS MANAGER

1. She/he should determine the capital budget of the hospital.
2. She/he should manage the liquid resources.
3. She/he should establish the credit policy of the hospital.
4. The level of inventories should be controlled in various departments.
5. She/he should establish the financial leverage.

6. She/he should negotiate and develop relationship with various suppliers of capital to obtain finance and good products.
7. She/he should maintain relationship with bankers.
8. Cash management is one of the important duties of finance manager.
9. She/he should maintain and control financial/management accounting.
10. She/he should conduct Internal audit of all the departments.
11. Periodical costing of the departments especially diagnostic department should be done.
12. Statutory payments should be paid on due dates (licenses, taxes, etc).
13. Based on the availability of funds, financial approval should be given for purchase of hospital equipments and other assets.
14. She/he should prepare projected Income and expenditure and balance sheet of the hospital for future years to understand the trend of the financial position of the hospital and also to submit the same to the Banks for loans.

PROJECT REPORT

It is essential to prepare a project report for hospital before starting a hospital or for the purpose of submitting the same to the banks for financial assistance or in case of hospital expansion.

To prepare a project report for hospital the following points should be discussed in detail:

1. The top management should decide and have a clear policy regarding the proposed facilities of the hospital. These include various specialty services like:
   a. General medicine
   b. General surgery
   c. Cardiology
   d. Pediatrics
   e. Dental
   f. Dermatology, etc.
   g. Clinical laboratories
   h. Radiology
   i. Ultrasound and other diagnostic facilities.
2. Break-up of beds
   The details of beds allotted to each specialty and each category of beds should be finalized as follows.

Specialty wise:

a. General medicine
b. General surgery
c. Cardiology
d. Gastroenterology
e. Ophthalmology
f. Obstetrics and gynecology
g. Orthopedics
h. ICU/IMCU
i. Others.

Categorywise:

- General ward (non-air conditioner)
- General ward air conditioner
- Semi private non-air conditioner
- Semi private air conditioner
- Private (single) air conditioner
- Private non-air conditioner
- Deluxe
- VIP suite/super deluxe
- ICU/Emergency ward
- Pediatric intensive care unit
- Newborn intensive care unit
- Casualty
- Isolation ward
- Triage.

3. Diagnostic services
4. Support services
5. Emergency services
6. Administrative services
7. Major equipments to be purchase (a) Medical (b) Service.
8. Type of building and allotment of departments and its location (Key plan)
9. Organization structure and the salary structure for executors and other Management staff
10. Revenue assumption
11. Expenditure assumption.

PROJECT COST AND MEANS OF FINANCING

Project cost

S. Number	Description	Rupees in lacs
1.	Land and development cost	xxx
2.	Building cost	xxx
3.	Engineering services	xxx
4.	Hospital services	xxx
5.	Hospital furniture and fabrication	xxx
6.	Administrative services	xxx
7.	Medical equipments and instruments	xxx
8.	Preliminary and preoperative expenses	xxx
9.	Provision for contingencies	xxx
10.	Margin money on working capital	xxx
	Total	XXXXX

Means of financing

1.	Share capital	xxx
2.	Promoters contribution	xxx
3.	public issue	xxx
4.	Term loans from banks	xxx
5.	Term loans from others	xxx
	Total	XXXX

DETAILS OF PROJECT COST

1. Land and development cost
   a. Land cost including registration and legal charges
   b. Development cost including leveling of land, boundary walls, internal roads, drainage facilities, parking and land scraping, etc.
2. Building cost
   a. Hospital buildings civil construction cost, internal plumbing work, pump house, underground tanks/sumps
   b. Architects fees.
3. Engineering services
   a. Electrical works
   b. Transformers
   c. Generator sets
   d. Air conditioning
   e. Lifts–patients and service
   f. Communication system like EPABX, CCTV, nurse calling system, public address system, etc.

4. Hospital services
   a. Medical gases and vacuum pipeline manifold, central vacuum and alarm system, outlet points, etc.
   b. Hospital kitchen, including cookers, fryers, burners, appliances, refrigerators, deep freezers, racks, tables and trolleys, cooking gas pipe line, utensils, etc.
   c. Sterile supply: including washers. disinfectors, autoclaves, oven, racks, tables and trolleys, etc.
   d. Hospital laundry system
      i. Washing machine (industrial)
      ii. Squeezing machines
      iii. Drying machine
      iv. Ironing equipments.
   e. Computers
   f. Biomedical waste disposal system
      i. Sewage cleaning tank
      ii. Incinerator.
   g. Ambulance/transport
   h. Hospital mortuary.
5. Hospital furniture and fabricators
   a. Medical furniture, including beds, lockers, stools, tables, trolleys, wheel chairs, etc.
   b. Interiors
   c. Hospital fabrications, including counters, cabinets, shelves, and desks, etc.
   d. Color TVs/refrigerators and other accessories
6. Administrative services
   a. Computers, photocopies, typewriters, printers, cash registers, and other office automation machine
   b. Wireless and intercom, etc.
7. Medical equipments and instruments
   a. ICU equipments
   b. Operation theater equipments/instruments
   c. Diagnostic equipment
   d. Other medical equipment.
8. Preliminary and preoperative expenses
   a. Expenses during implementation period; includes salaries, training, travel expenses, etc.

   b. Interest and commitment charges on term loans
   c. Brokerage commissions, advertisement and stationary expenses
   d. Consultancy fees.
9. Provision for contingencies
   a. Based on the size of the project and the volume of transaction the percentage of the total cost of the above services.
10. Margin money for working capital
   a. Margin money requiring for working capital should be decided and mentioned in this column.

CALCULATION OF EXPECTED REVENUE

The major share of revenue to the hospital is from outpatient department, inpatients, diagnostic services and pharmacy.

The income from outpatient department can be calculated as mentioned below:

1. OPD revenue

   Average working days of OPD is around 300 days

   A. Registration charges = Number of patients per day × Registration charges per patient

   B. Doctors fees = Number of patients per day × fee per patient (hospital share)

   Total OPD revenue = A + B

2. Inpatients

   Bed charges include room rent, housekeeping charges and nursing charge to calculate bed charges the following table has to be prepaid

Type of Receipts Accommodation per day	Number of beds	Charges per day	Revenue per day	% of occupancy	Total
General bed	50	500	25000	60	15000
Single air conditioner	20	1000	20000	50	10000
Receipts per day					25000

   C. Total revenue from bed charges per annum = Receipts per day × 365

3. Income from diagnostic services

The income from imaging services and other diagnostic services can be calculated as mentioned below:

X-ray department

Working days	= 365 days
Number of patients expected per day	= a
Charges per test per patient	= b
Total revenue of the department	= a × b × 365 days

The revenue from other departments can also be calculated in a similar manner.

In addition to the above revenue, the hospital will gets income from other procedures and services rendered to the patients. While calculating the cost of each test and bed charges, it is very essential to calculate the breakeven analysis.

Preparation of financial statements like funds flow statement, income and expenditure account, balance sheet, debt service coverage ratio, break even analysis, etc. it is done in other organization.

The financial accounting system is similar to the other business organization.

The management has to decide on running a pharmacy in the hospital. Whether the pharmacy division is an independent unit or a part of hospital management. Secondly the maintenance of accounts, whether the purchases and sales of medicines should be taken into hospital expenditure and income side of the P and L account.

If pharmacy is an independent unit of the same management, the accounts should be maintained separately. The Net profit of pharmacy can be shown in P and L air conditioner of the hospital. Around 30% of the hospital revenues are from pharmacy sales. The second largest contribution to the hospital is from clinical laboratory and other diagnostic services.

Though the bed charges are the major heads of income, 90% of the income generated through bed charges is utilized for day today running of the hospital as operational and administrative overheads.

The approximate requirements to start a hospital of 100 beds.

Land cost and area depends upon the locality, city and market price.

Category	*Detail*
Land	Depends upon the locality
Building	45000 sqft needed
Staff	300 persons
Project cost	Ten crores without land cost
Car parking	Extra
For supporting services	As per the policy of the organization

It may vary from project to project depends upon the type of construction, interiors, number of operation theaters, equipments, and customer segment.

CHAPTER 23

Facility Management

IMPORTANCE OF FACILITIES MANAGEMENT IN HOSPITALS

In a multispecialty hospital apart from medical services, general administration, financial management and personnel management, the facility management is equally important. It mainly deals with cleaning and maintenance of hospital, procurement of materials, including drugs and equipments, biomedical waste management, pest control, toilets and wash room, etc.

PROCUREMENT AND MANAGEMENT OF MATERIALS

Improving procurement and management activities of hospitals, such as, supply of drugs and equipments, clinical unit budgets and management, changing staffing levels and mix, making more efficient use of facilities, reducing inappropriate use of drugs, health services and diagnostic tests, performance measurement and many other related activities.

BUILDING MAINTENANCE

Air conditioner and ventilation are the most important facilities to maintain in hospitals. Apart from these two, some of other services are also important. They are:

High and low voltage electrical supplies, generator back-up power, UPS, lighting, water treatment monitoring, cooling towers, drainage/plumbing, chlorination of water systems, load shedding, lifts, fire alarms, sprinkler systems, access systems, automatic entry barriers, building management systems, portable appliance testing, thermal imaging, heating and humidity, etc.

BIOMEDICAL WASTE MANAGEMENT

Services in this area include clinical waste, clinical waste bins, clinical waste bags, clinical washroom products, theater bins, dental waste, amalgam separation and dental waste containers, etc.

MAINTENANCE OF IT EQUIPMENTS

This includes services like, IT hygiene and cleaning services including the cleaning of telephones, computers, server rooms, fax machines, photocopiers, ATMs, chip and pin machines, etc.

PEST CONTROL

Services included are rat control, mouse control, fly control, bed bug control, bird control, wasp and hornet control, cockroach control, etc.

MAINTENANCE OF WASHROOMS AND TOILET HYGIENE

The services included are, air freshener and air purification, urinal hygiene, toilet hygiene, washroom vending, feminine hygiene, handwashing and drying, premium product range and washroom supplies.

Maintenance of hospitals is a very strenuous task, which may prove very stressful and costly for the hospital management. In these cases opting for facility management is wise, as it covers all the functions of a hospital.

STRATEGIES FOR THE SUCCESS OF FACILITY MANAGEMENT

Since the past decade facility management has seen great progress. With lots of areas still left to improve, the new quality systems in areas of facility management operations and maintenance are found to produce great rewards. For facility management to be successful, there are few basic strategies which are to be adopted compulsorily. They are:

- Preplanning of work activities and pre-establishing critical-to-quality standards
- Creating work teams which are self directeds
- Effective management of materials
- Right communication and collaboration with customers and stakeholders.

In addition to these basic strategies, many new strategies suiting to the present modern conditions are designed making the facility management preferable at any point of time.

IMPORTANCE OF AIR CONDITIONERS, AIR PURIFIERS, AND VENTILATION SYSTEMS FOR HOSPITALS

Hospital air conditioning is more important because these days proper air conditioning has also become a factor in patient therapy and in some cases controlled environment provides more rapid physical improvement as the growth of many disease causing organisms is influenced by the surrounding temperature. Hence, proper air conditioning is found to play an important role in the prevention and treatment of diseases. Apart from controlled temperature, indoor air quality in the hospitals should also be maintained at the acceptable levels because there are large number of bacteria and virus spread in the hospital environment. Air purifiers and proper ventilation system help in improving the indoor air quality.

The benefits of having proper air conditioning system, air purifiers and ventilation systems in the hospitals are many as they:

- Restrict the movement of air between the various departments of the hospital
- Help in the dilution and removal of contaminants, which are in the form of airborne microorganisms, viruses, odor, hazardous chemicals and radioactive substances with ventilation and filteration
- Provide different types of temperature and humidity required for various areas in the hospital
- Help in controlling the environmental conditions, quality and circulation of the air
- Help patients with some diseases, such as thyrotoxicosis who cannot tolerate hot and humid conditions and in such cases, a cool and dry environment favors the loss of heat by radiation and skin evaporation which may save the life of a patient
- Help preventing dry conditions which may prove hazardous to the ill and debilitated persons, contributing to secondary infection
- reduce operational costs and maintenance costs for a hospital.

Designing of an energy efficient air conditioning system by a hospital according to its needs and best international practices, delivers a high quality product that is heath safe.

VITAL ASPECTS OF FACILITY MANAGEMENT WHICH LEAD TO PATIENT SAFETY

- Compliance to rules, regulations, laws and byelaws, licenses, certifications and registrations which are checks that limit the risk associated with a professional activity

- Compliance reduces the chances of potential damage that ignorance can cause
- Building safety codes, fire safety rules, drug license, radiation protection rules, AERB guidelines, laws applicable for medical gases, electrical safety, lifts and patient and human rights are some of the aspects without which any Health care facility cannot be declared safe
- "Compliance should be for the safety of patient and not just for a legal formality" A well documented and operational breakdown plan for corrective and preventive maintenance of all equipment particularly life saving equipment
- Ensuring back up for power, medical gases, spare supply and methodic equipment Management planning ensures patient safety. Calibration of machines saves the patient from misdiagnosis
- Log books record the functions of the machines which is very essential
- Adequate training of staff in using the equipment—saves the patient and saves the equipment. Renovations in a healthcare facility invariably compromises patient safety. Plans to put special precautions during renovations helps in maintaining patient safety
- Heating, Ventilation and Air Conditioning (HVAC) systems to be installed considering the possibility of spread of infection through HVAC due to faulty design and incomplete planning
- Building materials used for the facility to be non used for the facility to be nontoxic, fire toxic, fire resistant and meeting safety levels of material constituents
- Protocols should be in place for accidental exposure to any such material
- Equipment functioning forms an integral part of surgical safety checklist Thus patient safety derived out of usage of standard checklists depends upon error free equipment management and subsequent engineering support—both of which are elements of facility management
- Hygiene plan for the facility and disinfection protocol- for critical, semi-critical and noncritical items
- Layout, floor plans, and fire escape routes- they are not just pictures that we put on the walls but life line in emergencies
- Space allocation for various activities in a healthcare facility should be as per international or national standards. They help us in making our environment risk free and safe
- Inspection of waste disposal methods, water storage systems, ignition machinery, duct and pipeline maintenance are some areas which get low priority but have highest importance because cables and pipelines are arteries and veins of a hospital

- Agents ensures safe treatment and correct values of fluoride, heavy metals and salts protects the machines from corrosion
- Electrical back up with correct load estimation. LT (Low-tension) and HT (High-tension) supply disintegration keeps connections safe and protects patients who are on support of biomedical equipment
- Back up "Gas Bank" to provide medical gases when main supply fails
- Auto alarm systems and output detectors for all medical gases, vacuum and compressed air supplies
- *Key principles*—prevention, protection and life safety detection system with adequate technology application—autosprinkler systems, i-buildings fire calls, exit plans, bomb threat Management, and terrorist attack neutralizing plan
- Training of staff, drills and application of hospital emergency codes forms the most crucial aspect of handling any emergency
- Chemical, biological, radiological and nuclear (CBRN) disaster protocols-with separate triage areas so as to keep other patients safe
- Healthcare institutions handle a lot of hazardous material for a number of diagnostic and therapeutic activities. Their usage demands strict protocols, alertness and post-usage containment
- Small activity like biomedical waste management can actually enhance patient safety
- Patient safety cycle constitutes right usage, right way of usage and right disposal after use. It also includes right disposal of human waste after exposure to radiological matter
- Facility management has direct impact on hospital infection rate
- Housekeeping and hygiene have greatest impact on HAI (Healthcare associated infection) rates
- Surveillance of facility shows whether the infection is under permissible limits or not
- Infection control protocols needs to be an integral part of patient safety
- Patient safety is incomplete without fool proof planning and functioning of CSSD
- Technology brings in the possibility of hand-hygiene sensors and laser particle counters which could be installed at the entrances of the critical areas, thus helping a healthcare worker, know whether he or she is safe to entre and deliver care
- Patient identification using finger printing assures that the unique identification of patient is tallied with the various processes that a patient becomes a part of the organization

- Similarly, safety of high alert medications could be achieved if the medications and dozes are bar coded as per prescription and radiofrequency ID or magnetic bar coding is incorporated with medication management
- Green hospitals are safer hospitals due to high degree of patient environment protection that they provide. How many hospitals have railing in hospitals toilets, how many hospitals have beds with railing and how many wards have patient alarm call systems?
- A risk free stay must be given to inpatients. Provision of belts is one of the most inexpensive facilities that could be provided to stretcher, trolleys, and patient transport systems
- Detectors could be helpful in letting care givers know if the patient is crossing the physical limits of stretchers, beds, trolleys and can greatly reduce patient falls
- Internal and external disasters bring in an increased workload and a crunch of existing resources
- Disease outbreak management plan and external disaster management plans not only helps in providing care to the victims of such disasters but also protects the other patients from unsafe situations
- Earmarking of treatment areas with well planned air circulation systems, storages space, human resources planning and sanitation system planning for internal and external disasters are scientific steps to enhance patient safety
- All national and international standards places extreme importance to facility management and safety and an entire chapter is dedicated to enhance patient safety by improving facility management
- NABH recommends 9 standards and 43 objective elements for facility management and safety.

ROLES OF FACILITY MANAGERS FOR MANAGING ACTIVITIES

Facility management is an important sector that is involved in the co ordination of all business support activities. The facility management operators rely on various tools and equipment for business support activities that require the need for innovation and care in a wide range of facilities provided in commercial buildings such as hospitals, hotels, shopping malls, educational institutions, residential complexes, etc.

Facility manager is a person who plays an important role in managing facilities. He is also considered as a care taker of different premises around the environment in which people normally live or an infrastructure that provides a good quality of the facilities for the people to live in.

Facility managers have to operate at two levels—strategic and operational levels. In the first level, facility managers must inform their owners about the impact of their decisions regarding the provision of space and services. In the next level, facility manager's role is to provide and ensure proper operations of a building that creates an optimal, safe and cost effective environment in all aspects of a building. This is accomplished by managing and following some activities that are to be done by facility managers.

Their functions include providing health and safety services at local, State and national buildings, fire safety, housekeeping, gardening, cleaning, landscaping, security, facade maintenance, waste management and pest control. They are also supposed to take care of maintaining the power generation and air conditioning equipment, periodic testing and inspections of electrical portable equipment, work equipment and lift equipment, providing security and hospitality services within the buildings.

The facility mangers provide support and improve the effectiveness of the primary activities of a building by maintaining and developing the activities in various premises.

CHAPTER 24

Committees in Hospitals

The regulatory agency like Quality Council of India or Joint Council of India has prescribed regular standing committees for multi specialty hospitals. These committees are necessary in hospital administration in formulation of policies, coordination and monitoring wide activities of the hospital which are considered critical in the delivery of quality healthcare services.

These committees are divided into two types:

1. Committees dealing with hospital administrative matters
2. Committees dealing with medical matters.

Committees dealing with administrative matters.

ADMINISTRATIVE COMMITTEES

Executive Committee	
Members of the committee	Directors/trustees, CEO, president or vice-president and general managers.
Objects of the committee	To make policy decisions to improve the standards of the hospital. To improve the hospital infrastructure
Areas of responsibility	Quality services and organizational direction.
Output expected	Effective and efficient governance policies, decision-making andover sight producing quality service and financial stability.

Management Committee	
Members of the committee	Management staff and administrator
Objects of the committee	To execute the policies defined in executive committee. To review the day-to-day administration of the hospital. To review the facilities provided to patients—manpower planning.
Area of responsibility	Quality services and operational management.
Output expected	Effective and efficient operational strategies producing quality service and financial stability.

Committee on Medical Services	
Members of the committee	Medical superintendent, coordinator, hospital administrator, representative of all disciplines and nursing representative.
Objects of the committee	To monitor services rendered by doctors. To discuss the complaints/suggestion given by patients regarding medical services.
Areas of responsibility	Quality medical services rendered by physicians.
Output expected	Quality medical services.

Ethics Committee	
Members of the committee	One medical professional from outside hospital CEO and administrator, research doctors and physicians, advocate (legal), social worker, philanthropists, etc.
Objects of the committee	Study of drug trial, DNB project reports.
Areas of responsibility	Bioethical matters in patient care.
Output expected	Quality management system on bioethical matters in patients care.

Purchase Committee	
Members of the committee	End user, director, finance and accounts officer.
Objects of the committee	Review purchases—equipments, Maintenance, material, housekeeping items, etc.
Areas of responsibility	Quality purchases and budget allocation.
Output expected	Better control on purchases and inventory.

COMMITTEES DEALING WITH PATIENT CARE, QUALITY MEDICAL SERVICES, AND BIOMEDICAL WASTAGE

1. Safety and Risk Management Committee
2. Pharmacotherapeutic Committee
3. Hospital Infection Control Committee
4. Quality Assurance Committee
5. Medical Audit Committee
6. Blood Transfusion Committee
7. Cardiopulmonary Resuscitation Committee
8. Prevention of Sexual Harassment Committee
9. Death Audit Committee.

Safety and Risk Management Committee	
Members of the committee	Facility management staffs, clinicians, administrators, nursing head and paramedical staff, CEO, CMO.
Objectives of the committee	Sentinal events.
Area of responsibility	Monitoring and improving safety measures.
Output expected	Safety of patients, staff, doctors, Infrastructure.

Pharmacotherapeutic Committee	
Members of the committee	Major clinical department heads, administrator.
Objectives of the committee	Advance drug reaction drug formulary book.
Area of responsibility	Clinical pharmacist report, purchase of mew drugs.
Output expected	Quality management system on purchase, storage.

Hospital Infection Control Committee	
Members of the committee	Hospital administrator, Microbiologist physician services and if necessary include various departments' in charges as invitees
Objectives of the committee	Hand hygiene practice. Surveillance, Fumigation reports CAUTI, DVT, UTI Communicable disease Antibiotic policy Needle stick injury report HIC training program Safety and infection controlpractice in high risk areas Nonavailability of drugs Out breaks in hospital Sterilization recall
Ares of responsibility	Control of hospital associated (acquired) infection
Output expected	Hospital associated infection
Abbreviations	VAP—ventilator associated pneumonia SSI—surgical site infection CAUTI—catheter associated urinary tract infection DVT—deep vein thrombosis UTI—urinary tract infection.

Quality Assurance Committee	
Members of the committee	Representation from management,
Objectives of the committee	Key indicator (quality indicator) Employee satisfaction
Area of responsibility	Quality services and quality management
Output expected	Quality management system in place

Medical Audit Committee	
Members of the committee	Medical superintendent, co-ordinator hosptial, administrator, representative of all disciplines and nursing representative
Objectives of the committee	Case sheet audit, clinic audit criteria for selection of case sheet
Area of responsibility	Ensure proper care to patients
Output expected	Outcome in-patient care, such as mortality

Blood Transfusion Committee	
Members of the committee	Blood transfusion office, CMO, administration Surgery, nursing supdt, physicians, lab, inc.
Objectives of the committee	Blood transfusion reactions Rectification Action taken to reduce blood transfusion reaction Discussion to improve blood andblood products Quality management system on infection control
Area of responsibility	Blood transfusion
Output expected	Quality management system in blood transfusion.

Cardiopulmonary Resuscitation Committee	
Members of the committee	Physicians, anesthetist and nurses, code blue team (ACLS/BLS trained)
Objectives of the committee	CPR events Reports on CPR events Code blue events
Area of responsibility	Training program in BLS and ACLS
Output expected	More number of survivals through CPR procedure

Prevention of Sexual Harassment Committee	
Members of the committee	Maximum lady members, CMO, HR manager, nursing supervisors, social worker, etc.
Objectives of the committee	Any complaints received from the lady staff
Area of responsibility	prevention of sexual harassment in the organization
Output expected	Provide safety and security to female staff.

Death Audit Committee	
Members of the committee	Medical superintendent, concern doctors,
Objectives of the committee	Selection of case sheet
Area of responsibility	Outcome in patient care, such as mortality
Output expected	Acceptable mortality, morbidity and unnecessary operation rate.

The main objects of these committees are to fulfill the tasks effectively and efficiently which will lead to quality outcome and excellent results with nil complaints from the patients.

The important functions of these committees are:

a. Formulating policies
b. Coordination
c. Monitoring the hospital wide activities on specified areas of responsibility.

These committees also provide proper training and education to respective staff to promote goal achievement.

TYPES OF COMMITTEE MEMBERS

Type	*Function*	*Attendance*	*Membership*	*Tenure*
Regular	Fulfill prescribed tasks	Regular	Appointed	One year subject to renewal
Ad hoc	To assist regular members	As needed	As per the invitation by regular members	One year subject to renewal
Ex-officio	Advise	As needed	Invited or designated	One year subject to renewal

With regards to the committee meetings the following document and details of action taken report should be maintained:

1. Minutes of the meetings.
2. Review of points in previous meeting.
3. Performance reports or action taken reports.
4. Preventive measures taken.
5. Inter office communication.
6. Management review report—once a year.

TIPS FOR EFFECTIVE FUNCTIONING OF COMMITTEES

1. Selection of objectives.
2. Selection of members who are dedicated and interested for the development of the hospital.
3. Healthy discussions and allowing open discussion without any reservations or prejudice.
4. Decision making keeping in view the over all objectives of the hospital.
5. Implementation of decisions taken in committee.
6. Inform action taken report to the members.
7. Review of points which are not closed.
8. Closer of points.
9. Preventive measures without concentrating only on complaints and suggestions.
10. Effective interoffice communication.

CHAPTER 25

Insurance Help Desk

Functions of this department are:

- To coordinate with the insurance companies and patients regarding cash less treatment.
- To help patients in sending preauthorization forms to the insurance patients
- To coordinate with the billing section in preparation of final bills for TPA patients.
- To clarify the doubts of patients regarding cash less treatment.

PROCEDURE

At the time of admission a patient or attendant should inform to the receptionist about the Mediclaim card number and relation to the card holder. The Receptionist will put the stamp with the particulars of insurance company on the case sheet.

After the admission of patient or before admission either patient or attendant will go to the TPA help desk for filling necessary forms.

After initial assessment the officer in TPA help desk will fill pre-authorization forms with the help of billing staff and the ward doctor.

In preauthorization form the following details will be mentioned:

a. Name of the patient
b. Name of the hospital
c. Insurance ID number
d. Corporate name/employee code
e. Present complaints
f. Provisional diagnosis
g. Proposed treatment plan

h. Medical history of patient
i. Admission details
j. Approximate cost of treatment
k. Signature of treating doctor.

After filling the columns in pre-authorization form it will be sent through e-mail to the concern insurance company by the TPA help desk officer.

Copies of the ID proof of patient, i.e. ID card issued by the insurance companies should be produced by the patient to TPA help desk to process the application for cashless treatment.

The insurance company will take 4–6 hours to reply for pre authorization application.

If the insurance company is satisfied with the particulars mentioned in pre authorization form, it will sanction the limit for cash less treatment based on the policy of the card holder.

The patient is eligible for treatment on cashless basis up to the limit mentioned in the approval. The balance amount should be paid by the patient.

When a hospital bill exceeds the sanctioned limit, the officer in TPA help desk will send a requisition to the insurance company for enhancement of limit along with the copy of the bill.

If the insurance company is satisfied with the excess of bill amount and reason for extradays stay in hospital it will send a revised approval either for full amount or a part of bill amount based on the eligibility of the insured.

Sometimes, the insurance companies may ask for more details or clarifications for queries raised by their medical officer.

After submitting the details, the insurance company may or may not give approval for cash less treatments.

Since the insurance company does not give any reason for refusal for cash less treatment hospitals are facing lot of problems with patients. Patients will be under the impression that they get free treatment in the hospital once they show their insurance ID card.

DUTIES AND RESPONSIBILITIES OF A FRONT OFFICER IN TPA HELP DESK

1. He should have a complete knowledge about the insurance companies, procedure to get approval.
2. He should know the terms and conditions of each and every insurance company a functioning under IRDA.

Delay may also be due to nonavailability of insurance details of patients. Sometimes, after two to three days of admission, the patient or his attendant might inform the billing section that he has got an insurance coverage. After that the process of getting approval for cashless treatment starts.

The clear systems, communications and awareness of the procedures among the card holder makes the process simple and effective for getting claims early.

GUIDELINES TO TPA (INSURANCE) PATIENTS

1. If any patient wanted to take treatment under cashless treatment he/she should submit the insurance particulars to the TPA help desk within 24 hours from the time of admission, failing which the management is not responsible for any refusal of claim or approval by the insurance companies.
2. The insured person should bring the insurance ID card/policy copy at the time of admission and produce a Xerox copy of the same subsequently in the TPA help Desk.
3. The insured person or insured person representatives, when he/she is unable to personally communicate due to medical condition should send a request for hospitalization to the insurance company.
4. The credit facility will be given to the insured person only after receiving the approval letter from the insurance company with the entitlement of available benefits.
5. In case of emergencies, insured persons will be admitted on the identity established through ID cards.
6. The credit facilities will be given up to the sanctioned amount mentioned in the approval letter.
7. The insured person shall be given an indemnity letter to the hospital at the time of admission.
8. Kindly make sure that the dully filled pre-authorization form will be sent back to the TPA Help desk by the ward incharge.
9. The insured person is not eligible for claim on credit facility for the treatment of the pre-existing disease as per the insurance policy.
10. Any suppression of facts regarding the pre-existing disease at the time of admission or during the time of treatment, the insured person is liable for payment of hospital bills.
11. The insured person shall pay the cost of non-medical items such as special attender charges, telephone, snacks, food, beverages, etc. directly to the hospital for which some amount should be paid by the patient

as advance at the time of admission. The balance amount will be refunded after adjusting the disallowed items in the final bill.

12. At the time of discharge, patient should pay if the patient avails the following facilities.
    (a) Excess room rent and nursing charges for higher category stay
    (b) Room rent and nursing charges if the Room is occupied by the attendant
    (c) Extra attendant charges as per rules of the hospital.
13. In case the insurance company fails to send the approval letter before discharge the insured person shall make the payment to the hospital at the time of discharge and claim reimbursement as per his eligibility.
14. If the insurance company refuses the claim after discharges, the insured person has to settle the hospital bill amount as per the indemnity letter signed by the insured perons or his/her representatives.
15. Only one TPA insurance card will be accepted for one hospitalization. The amount cannot be split and send to different TPA companies for the same admission. The authorized amount is less than the bill amount; the balance amount should be paid by the patient at the time of discharge.
16. The approval for cashless treatment, eligibility amount, co-payment, disallowed things for cashless treatment will be based on the terms and conditions mentioned in the final approval letter by the company.
17. Some of the insurance companies insist on further approval for final bill amount though the initial approval for cashless treatment is given. In such cases it will take minimum of 6 to 8 hours to get the final approval after the confirmation of discharge by the consultant.
18. If the patient is particular about getting discharge before final approval, he has to pay the total bill amount. This amount will be refunded to him/her once the final approval is received from the insurance companies after deducting the approval amount.
19. For other insurance patients the difference amount of bill amount and approval amount will be collected at the time of discharge, if the patient wanted to get discharge before the approval of enhancement request. The same will be refunded if the hospital receive the approval for final bill amount.
20. In case of denial of cashless treatment by the insurance company for any reason the patient has to pay full bill amount at the time of discharge.
21. As per the instructions given by the insurance companies the patient is eligible for room rent and nursing charges put together equivalent

of 1% of sum insured by the insurer or as mentioned in the approval letter.

22. For individual policy other than the corporate companies the Nursing charges are not eligible and the same should be paid by the patient.
23. In case of denial by the Insurance companies, the help desk can only help the patient to send the reconsideration letter to the insurance companies for approval and the management is not responsible for any denial.
24. Since most of the insurance companies are not working on Sundays, National Holidays, the management cannot send the pre-authorization form or confirmation form.
25. If any patient wants to get discharge on these days he has to pay the final bill amount and he/she can either claim reimbursement from the company or he/she will be refunded the bill amount once the approval is received by the hospital from the insurance companies.
26. If patient is admitted under surgical package he is eligible as per the package charges if there is any difference of package amount due to more number of days stay or occupied the higher category of room than the eligible category room it should be paid by the patient at the time of discharge.

CHAPTER 26

Communication

Good medical care depends upon effective communication between patients and providers. Ineffective communication can lead to improper diagnosis and delayed or improper medical treatment. Effective communication with persons who have limited English proficiency, as well as persons who are deaf or hard-of-hearing, often requires interpreters or other services. Many hospitals are actively taking steps to address these needs. However, hospitals face increasing challenges to meet the communication needs of an increasingly diverse population. Though the effective communication between patients and providers helps get better patient satisfaction, inadequate communication between management and employees cause misunderstanding, confusion and, occasionally, total chaos. On the other hand, proper communication can pave the way for better relations, greater job satisfaction on account of clarity about job requirements and organizational goals, better cooperation, fostering attitudes necessary for motivation, etc.

NATURE AND SCOPE OF COMMUNICATION

Communication is the process of passing messages from one person to another. The use of the word 'mind' is intended to imply the importance of conveying facts, ideas, emotions, opinions and all other types of instructions in such a way that they can be understood by the person receiving them. A significant point about communication is that it always involves two people—a sender and a receiver.

PURPOSE OF COMMUNICATION

Results are achieved in an organization through the process of communication. If there is a proper system of communication in an organization, there will not be any misunderstanding and confusion. Communication is needed not only by the managerial staff for discharging their duties efficiently, but also by the lowest employees to listen to the instructions of their supervisors and to perform their duties sincerely. Proper communication is needed at every step and serves several purposes.

A good communication system results in better patient-care and higher job satisfaction through better team-work.

IMPORTANCE OF COMMUNICATION IN HOSPITALS

On the surface, communication appears to be a simple concept within health care. Patients talk to doctors, nurses, and staff members. Doctors explain treatment options to patients. However, many obstacles often get in the way of understandable, quality communication. A lack of quality communication limits the quality of service that can be provided to the patient. Some of these issues are rooted within health care system design, while others are the result of inappropriate services provided to patients. Communication limitations often make the patients' visits frustrating and unpleasant.

Consider a typical hospital inpatient visit. Upon arrival, a patient completes paperwork, talks to various staff about where to go and what to do, talks to physicians about his ailments, and talks to a number of nurses about the procedures of the hospital. These interactions might creat an unwanted confusion in the patients in their relation with the health care providers. It should be noted that patients have special characteristics which differ them from a regular customer who wants to receive a service. They are not in their best physical or mental condition, making communication with this type of customer unique. Although it is a common belief that physicians talking to patients reduce patient anxiety and increases patient satisfaction, there is no indication that talking to multiple health care providers would also be beneficial. Moreover, it will create confusion in the minds of patients/ attendants.

POOR COMMUNICATION BETWEEN HEALTHCARE STAFF AND PATIENTS IN HOSPITAL

Nearly half of patients are given no details about the side effects of the medicines they are given:

Few members of the healthcare team only confirm their identity prior to administering medication and prior to performing an operation or procedure.

Some patients' express that they had questions they would have liked to ask the members of their healthcare team but did not do so, due to fear of proper care and treatment.

The following procedures must be followed by healthcare providers while they attend on patients.

- Avoid discussing medical issues at patients' bed side ignoring the patients or the attendants.
- Avoid delaying admission due to lack of co ordination and communication between the departments.
- Communicate to patients regarding cancelation and rescheduling of operation/procedures.
- Encourage patients to express their views about the hospital services.
- Communicate to patients about the non availability of consultants and the reappointment date.

BARRIERS TO EFFECTIVE COMMUNICATION

Effective communication within hospitals depends on efficient patient care coordination, proper use of technology, and sound communication management procedures. Barriers to any of these can impede the effective transfer of information among hospital staff, good communication in the healthcare setting is becoming harder to achieve with complex technology, increased patient needs and lack of resources.

PATIENT CARE COORDINATION

Patient-centered communication allows doctors and nurses to reach populations entering hospitals from a variety of cultures and backgrounds. According to a communication barriers study non-English speaking patients often encounter inappropriate medical treatment and hospitalization because of the language barrier between patient and doctor. Hospitals often lack the time and money needed to initiate effective communication strategies, such as creating community advisory boards and recruiting diverse staff of healthcare workers.

HEALTH INFORMATION TECHNOLOGY

With advances in technology, hospital workers are becoming more reliant on high-tech devices and less on forms of written communication. Pagers, computers and cell phones keep doctors and nurses electronically connected, but more wiring can create more grievous errors. According to the National Center of Policy Analysis, health information systems can intensify problems when electronic medical records contain false information that is relied upon by hospital staff. A 2010 University of California study reported that the simple use of whiteboards and dry erase markers by bedside nurses were effective communication tools, not to be replaced by high-tech equipment.

COMMUNICATION MANAGEMENT PROCEDURES

Shorter hospital stays, higher nurse-to-patient ratios, and a hectic health-care environment have created gaps in communication and led a variety of healthcare organizations to suggest ways hospitals can improve communication practices.

BARRIERS TO EFFECTIVE COMMUNICATION BY NURSES

LANGUAGE BARRIERS

The possibility of miscommunication increases when the nurse and patient speak different languages. Idioms and frames of reference can carry shades of meaning in one language that may not exist in another. Mispronunciation or incorrect signing can mislead the provider or patient. A translator can improve the situation when a nurse who speaks the language is unavailable.

ETHNIC BARRIERS

Differences in ethnic background and mores can create communication problems. Societal expectations about the human body and its exposure to others can interfere with a nurse performing her duties and explaining follow-up care for a patient. What one culture considers a normal condition may camouflage illness. Learning about cultural differences can reduce many of these barriers.

STAFFING SHORTAGES

Effective communication takes time: time to determine the patient's condition, time to explain and educate, time to confirm that the patient understands. The shortage of nurses in many medical settings can lead to lack of time. Without enough nurses on staff, the amount of time available for each patient declines.

ASSUMPTIONS

A nurse who makes assumptions about a patient based on a case diagnosis risks missing important clues. Open-minded communication between patient and nurse permits better assessment and more accurate care plans.

DISTRACTIONS

Nurses in a medical facility care for multiple patients at a time, creating a situation ripe for distractions and interruptions. Situations outside the workplace also can create distractions. Effective communication requires committed attention, something nurses may find more difficult to give with the increasing demands on them.

MEDICAL JARGON

Nurses can intimidate or confuse patients with the use of medical jargon. This can be rectified by using common terms with a patient to simplify the conversation. Adding a simple "which is" explanation after a medical term can improve the patient's understanding.

HEALTH LITERACY BARRIERS

People with poor literacy skills are especially challenged by most health information. There is a huge disparity between how people receive and comprehend health information. Language and cultural barriers are linked with low health literacy.

EFFECTIVE COMMUNICATION

Effective communication is an important part of all of our lives, but never so much as when we are seeing a doctor. Effective communication in health care is critical for the correct diagnosis, correct care, effective treatment, legal processes and medical progress.

CORRECT DIAGNOSIS

Effective communication in the healthcare industry is incredibly important in aiding in the correct diagnosis of an individual's condition. It is very important that both the healthcare providers and the patient are very clear in what they say to one another. If the patient is unclear, inconsistent or limited in the information he provides regarding his symptoms and past experiences, the diagnosis the healthcare providers comes up with may be inaccurate, leading to mistreatment of the condition.

HISTORY

It is very important that the patient is very clear in communicating her medical history to healthcare professionals. Drug allergies, medical conditions, previous surgeries and illnesses can provide critical information to doctors and nurses while the patient is in the hospital. Failure to effectively communicate these parts of a medical history can put a patient's life at risk. For example, failure to mention an allergy to penicillin can cause a patient to go into an anaphylactic shock.

TREATMENT

Communication is a very crucial part of the treatment process. Healthcare professionals must effectively communicate instructions for medication and home treatment to the patient. A misunderstanding could result in an overdose or the worsening of the condition. Patients must ask questions about their treatment, if they are unclear about the instructions.

LEGAL PROCESSES

Effective communication is important for legal issues pertaining to treatment. A thorough understanding of diagnoses and treatments must be established before a healthcare professional can proceed. Documentation of all communications can become important should something go wrong. Documentation of the communication that has taken place can provide a defense for the hospital, or ammunition for the plaintiff.

MEDICAL PROGRESS

Communication is critical for advancing medical progress. Information gathered at a hospital or doctor's office can help track things like outbreaks of the flu or other communicable diseases. Information about the disease can help healthcare providers to stockpile certain medications in advance ultimately saving lives.

CHAPTER 27

Safety and Security

One of the important duties and responsibilities of the top management in formulating policies and procedures of hospital is regarding safety and security of (i) the patients, (ii) the staff, (iii) the attendants, (iv) the doctors, (v) the machines, and (vi) the infrastructure.

Each and every employee should follow the rules and regulations of the hospital and has to cooperate with the management in implementing various safety measures in the hospital; this can be achieved by participating in training programs.

Safety committee one of the important committees of a hospital, is constituted to monitor and to study of various safety measures to prevent accidents in the hospital premises

Many bold decisions are taken, to provide safety to the employees, the patients, the attendants, etc. by the representative from the top management as the chairperson of the committee. Some of the important functions of the committee is to discuss and go through the accident and incident reports, actions taken to prevent these incidents and accidents.

DEFINITION OF PATIENT SAFETY

Patient safety is a discipline in the healthcare sector that applies safety science methods toward the goal of achieving a trustworthy system of health-care delivery. Patient safety is also an attribute of healthcare systems; it minimizes the incidence and impact of, and maximizes recovery from, adverse events.

Patient safety is the avoidance, prevention, and amelioration of adverse outcomes or injuries stemming from the processes of health care.

These events include "errors," "deviations," and "accidents." Safety emerges from the interaction of the components of the system; it does not reside in a person, device or department. Improving safety depends on learning how safety emerges from the interactions of the components. Patient safety is a subset of healthcare quality.

The areas of patient safety include maintaining hygiene and safety of injections, blood, drugs, chemicals, transplants, clinical procedures, medical devices, immunization, etc.

GOALS

- To identify patients correctly
- To improve effective communication among care givers
- To improve the safety of the medications
- To reduce the risk of healthcare-associated infections
- To reconcile medications across the continuum of care
- To reduce the risk of patient harm resulting from falls
- To reduce the risk of influenza and pneumococcal disease in institutionalized elderly patients
- To reduce the risk of surgical fires
- To encourage patients' active involvement in their own care as a patient safety strategy
- To prevent healthcare-associated pressure like ulcers.

PATIENT SAFETY TIPS FOR HOSPITALS

Medical errors may occur in different health care settings, and those that happen in hospitals can have serious consequences. The agency for healthcare research and quality, which has sponsored hundreds of patient safety research and implementation projects, offers these 10 evidence-based tips to prevent adverse events from occurring in any hospital:

1. Prevent central line-associated bloodstream infections. Be vigilant preventing central line-associated bloodstream infections by taking five steps every time a central venous catheter is inserted:
   a. Washing your hands.
   b. Using full-barrier precautions.
   c. Cleaning the skin with chlorhexidine.
   d. Avoiding femoral lines, and
   e. Removing unnecessary lines.
   f. Taking these steps consistently will reduce this type of deadly healthcare-associated infection to zero.

2. Re-engineer hospital discharges. Reduce potentially preventable readmissions by assigning a staff member to work closely with patients and other staff to reconcile medications and schedule necessary follow up medical appointments. Create a simple, easy-to-understand discharge plan for each patient that contains a medication schedule, a record of all upcoming medical appointments, and names and phone numbers of whom to call if a problem arises.
3. Prevent venous thromboembolism. Eliminate hospital-acquired venous thromboembolism (VTE), the most common cause of preventable hospital deaths, by using an evidence-based guide to create a VTE protocol.
4. Educate patients about using blood thinners safely. Patients who have had surgery often leave the hospital with a new prescription for a blood thinner, such as Coumadin®, to keep them from developing dangerous blood clots. However, if used incorrectly, blood thinners can cause uncontrollable bleeding and are among the top causes of adverse drug events.
5. Limit shift durations for medical residents and other hospital staff if possible. Evidence shows that acute and chronically fatigued medical residents are more likely to make mistakes. Ensure that residents get ample sleep and adhere to 80-hour workweek limits. Residents who work 30-hour shifts should only treat patients for up to 16 hours and should have a 5-hour protected sleep period between 10 pm and 8 am.
6. Consider working with a patient safety organization. Report and share patient safety information with patient safety organizations (PSOs) to help others avoid preventable errors. By providing both privilege and confidentiality, PSOs create a secure environment where clinicians and health care organizations can use common formats to collect, aggregate, and analyze data that can improve quality by identifying and reducing the risks and hazards associated with patient care.
7. Use good hospital design principles. Follow evidence-based principles for hospital design to improve patient safety and quality. Prevent patient falls by providing well-designed patient rooms and bathrooms and creating decentralized nurses' stations that allow easy access to patients. Reduce infections by offering single bed rooms, improving air filtration systems, and providing multiple convenient locations for hand washing. Prevent medication errors by offering pharmacists well-lit, quiet, private spaces so they can fill prescriptions without distractions.
8. Measure the hospital's patient safety culture. Survey hospital staff to assess the facilities for patient safety culture. If the health system includes

nursing homes or ambulatory care medical groups, share culture surveys that are customized for those settings.

9. Build better teams and rapid response systems. Train hospital staff to communicate effectively as a team.
10. Insert chest tubes safely. Keep in mind the principles of UWET when inserting chest tubes. The easy-to-remember mnemonic is based on a universal protocol from the Joint Commission UMET means:
    a. Universal precautions (achieved by using sterile cap, mask, gown, and gloves)
    b. Wider skin prep
    c. Extensive draping
    d. Tray positioning.

PROBLEMS OF SECURITY IN HOSPITAL

It would be difficult to verify the bonafides of the visitors to the hospital as it is a public service organization. Like industries, the hospital cannot have a security checks for all the visitors, incoming or outgoing traffic. The entry cannot be restricted.

The visitors cannot be suspected. If the visitors are genuine and security person suspects it will badly reflect on patients sentiments. The outsiders who are not patients may act as patients or visitors and cheat the other patients/attendants.

SECURITY MEASURES

1. Out patients should be discouraged from loitering around or going into the inpatient wards. Uncontrolled movement of outpatients and visitors is not only a security risk but also a disturbance to inpatients and hospital routine work.
2. Hospital visiting hours should be observed strictly.
3. The attendant should be in possession of a pass issued by the hospital authorities.
4. Number of visitors should be restricted.
5. Only one attendant should be permitted to stay with the patient.
6. All staff entrusted with handling/custody of money and valuables will exercise the greatest care for their safety and be scrupulously honest in their accounting and disposal.
7. All cash and valuables collected by any individual during the course of the day will be handed over to the appropriate officer the same day for safe custody.

8. Patients should be discouraged from bringing large amount of money and valuables into the hospital.
9. Cash collections and the disbursal should always be conducted in an orderly manner. No one other than the cashier, her/his assistant should have access to the cash box.
10. All the staff should carry their personal valid identity card issued by the hospital authorities.
11. Proper gate pass system should be followed for the items going out or coming inside the hospital.

SAFETY MEASURES

1. Periodical checking of wheel chairs, stretches and other hospital furniture.
2. Provide safety belts for wheel chairs stretcher etc through which the patients are being transported from one ward to the other ward.
3. Provide uneven flooring in the wards or in the common areas where the movement of patients and visitors are more.
4. Provide anti skid material in the slope floor areas.
5. Provide grab bars in the ramps and in the toilets.
6. Periodical checking of Electrical points is essential to prevent short circuits.
7. Provide speed breakers on lengthy roads inside the hospital premises,and mark them in Yellow and White colours for recognition.
8. Provide proper sign boards wherever applicable like speed breakers, exit, emergency exit, fire emergency, etc.
9. Remove hanging wires, cables and periodical replacement of damaged cables, switch boards, loose fixtures sparkling appliances, etc.
10. Welding or any work with fire generation should not be permitted in the ward or departments without prior intimation to the safety manager. Safety manager should take proper precaution before undertaking such works.
11. Chemicals and oil substances should be stored in the main stores and other areas properly and avoid wooden cupboards for storage of such items.
12. Avoid excessive paper, plastic, cardboards, and wooden scrap in the wards and departments.
13. Usage of electrical gadgets other than the gadgets provided by the hospital should be prohibited.
14. Biomedical wastage like used bandages, cotton should be disposed off every day.

15. Fire fighting equipment should be provided in every ward and department in a prominent place. Proper training should be given to the employees for operating firefighting equipment.
16. Staff working in high risk areas should wear personal protective equipments (PPE) without fail.
17. Proper care should be taken while digging or demolishing buildings in case of modification or new structures to avoid the damage of cables and other electrical, telephone, computer CCTV cables, etc.
18. Empowering patients through education and informed consent.
19. Creating partnerships between providers and consumers to improve the quality of health care.
20. Improving work organization and services that are delivered including patient safety in medical and nursing curriculum.
21. Strengthening the numbers, distribution and skills of the workforce.
22. Moving patient safety beyond the hospital to community-level care.
23. Building patient safety into quality assurance programs.
24. Introducing non-punitive reporting and learning systems (careful and participatory surveillance).
25. Introducing simple, cost-effective patient safety measures that are in line with available human, physical and financial resources.
26. Improving infection control and waste management as components of quality assurance.
27. Strengthening accreditation, monitoring and supervision systems.
28. Strong leadership at the government and institutional levels and partners.
29. Other safety measures should be introduced in the areas of water, food and environmental sanitation including waste disposal and elimination of stray animals and maintaining building safety.

DUTIES OF SECURITY GUARDS

1. Guards should be posted at all strategic locations and at the main gate.
2. The security post should be located at the main gate.
3. Main gate should be manned round the clock. In other positions, authorities depending upon prevailing situation and hospital architecture should decide the trimmings.
4. Nursing hostel, if any, should be guarded round the clock.
5. The security guard is totally responsible for the security of the area assigned to him. She/He should not sleep while on duty. To start the duty, he should make sure that all the unoccupied rooms along with

its windows are securely locked. If any window or room is open, she/he should immediately inform the authorities (first to his supervisor if not to proper authority).

6. The guards on duty should not remain stationary during most of the time of their duty. They should patrol the area allotted to them and should be watchful of any unauthorized entry even by the hospital staff without valid reason. They can question any odd behavior or unauthorized entry.
7. The guards at the gates can guide the flow of traffic. The guards at the main gate can assist in parking of vehicles.
8. Main gate guards should not allow any hospital property to be taken out by anybody without proper gate pass.
9. Guards at nurse's hostel should ensure that hostel rules laid down by authorities are followed.
10. Guards should also assist in observation of general rules of economy.
11. In case of fire, minor or major, guards should follow a set line-of actions.

GUARDS AT OUT-GATE

1. One copy of the gate pass should be retained by the security at the gate and the gate security guard or in-charge security will sign other copies with date and time.
2. Whenever the material is received or returned at a gate pass, security should again sign other copies with date and time.
3. All gate passes should be numbered serially and should be file them and presented to the hospital managers. Returnable gate passes are time bound, and no entry allowed once data is over.
4. In case of duplicate gate pass as guards should check the signature of the hospital authorities.

DUTIES OF SECURITY OFFICER

1. The security officer is be in-charge of all security arrangements for the hospital.
2. He/she should adopt such measures as are necessary for the protection of men, material and information and implement them tactfully and discreetly. He/she should pay special attention to unhealthy or subversive influences of staff, movement of stores and material within the hospital and handling of cash and valuables.
3. The following are some of the vulnerable spots that have to be watched carefully:

a. Stores—receipt distribution and custody.
b. Laundry/disinfector/incinerator.
c. Cash collection and handling.
d. Unconscious patients/dead bodies—handling of cash and valuables.
e. Car park/scooter/cycle stands.
f. Misuse/abuse of services like telephones, water and electricity.

4. The security officer should divide the hospital area into convenient sectors and allot duties to his/her staff in these sectors. She/he will make periodical and surprise rounds to ensure that the staff are on the alert.
5. Minimum numbers of gates consistent with the efficient functioning of the hospital should be kept open and guards should be posted at required gates. Other gates should be kept locked and the keys deposited in the security office. After OPD hours only the 'IN' and 'OUT' gates of the OPD should be kept open. After OPD hours only the 'IN' gate of emergency should be open. This gate should be used for traffic of both ways.
6. Places like stores, main office, accounts office, nurse's hostel, and laundry are restricted to all except those on duty.
7. It is the duty of security officer to watch for unhealthy/subversive influence on the Staff of the hospital, which may lead to unrest, agitation, indiscipline and disturbances and take suitable measures promptly.
8. She/he should be able to effectively communicate to patients and other visitors.
9. She/he should be of sound mind and body and should be able to act sincerely, quickly and take decisions in cases of emergencies.
10. She/he should be aware of some legal concepts of providing security.
11. She/he should be able to physically remove an intruder, if required to do so.

DUTIES OF HOSPITAL FIRE OFFICER

In case of fire, the welfare and security officer, and his staff should cooperate with the hospital fire officer in the implementation of these orders. The duties of the hospital fire officer are as follows:

1. Preparation of plan for fires-fighting arrangements and its implementation.
2. Checking fire-fighting equipment periodically to ensure that all items are serviceable.
3. Training fire-fighting parties in their duties in fire-fighting, i.e. raising alarm, cordoning the scene of fire, salvage operations, fire-fighting with water and sand buckets, extinguishers and trailer pumps.

4. Keeping the fire orders up-to-date, giving them adequate publicity and ensuring that they are implemented.
5. Making sure that equipments for fire-fighting are located at all major and minor fire susceptible places within the hospital. The number and type of equipment at these stations will be as per local fire safety norms prescribed to obtain a "NOC" form the prescribed authorities.
6. Seeing that all emergency exit doors are not encroached upon and these doors have free access.
7. Seeing that all safety signs are properly displayed at all times.
8. To have proper knowledge of hazardous materials and should be able to operate fire-fighting equipments by himself.
9. The hospital fire officer should be well trained so that he can evacuate men and material when needed.

CHAPTER 28

Duties and Responsibilities of Hospital Staff

ACCOUNTS MANAGER

See page 154.

ADMINISTRATOR

See page 17.

BILLING STAFF

See page 199.

BIOMEDICAL ENGINEER

See page 101.

BLOOD BANK MEDICAL OFFICER

See page 81.

CHIEF FINANCE OFFICER

See page 154.

CHIEF MEDICAL OFFICER

See page 20.

CSSD TECHNICIAN

See page 202.

DIETICIAN

See page 58.

AMBULANCE DRIVER

See page 202.

FIRE OFFICER

See page 193.

HUMAN RESOURCE MANAGER

See page 143.

LINEN KEEPER

See page 199.

MAINTENANCE SUPERVISOR/FACILITY MANAGER

See page 205.

MALE NURSING ASSISTANT

See page 204.

MANIFOLD OPERATOR

See page 70.

MEDICAL RECORD OFFICER

See page 89.

NURSE

See page 25.

INFECTION CONTROL NURSE

See page 64.

OUTPATIENT DEPARTMENT RECEPTIONIST

See page 47.

OT IN-CHARGE

See page 78.

OT TECHNICIAN/NURSE

See page 79.

PHYSIOTHERAPIST

See page 206.

PERSONNEL MANAGER

See page 142.

PUBLIC RELATION OFFICERS

See page 204.

RECEPTIONIST

See page 197.

RESIDENT MEDICAL OFFICER

See page 24.

SANITARY TECHNICIAN

See page 201.

SECURITY OFFICER

See page 192.

SECURITY GUARDS

See page 191.

SWEEPERS

See page 201.

TPA HELP DESK FRONT OFFICER

See page 176.

WARD ASSISTANTS AND AYAHS

See page 203.

RECEPTIONIST (ALL SHIFTS)

Duties will depend upon the extent of the job description. Therefore, following duties should be taken as guidelines only:

1. No staff except the designated ones should be allowed to sit in the reception area.
2. All staff should enter the hospital in proper dress code.
3. Reception staff should not eat or drink at the counter.
4. All receptionists should greet a visitor, patient with a smiling face and repeated questioning of the visitor, and handle a visitor gently even if the visitor behaves indecently.

5. Every receptionist at the start of the shift has to make sure that the hospital's charge schedule is available. If the equipment is not in working condition, it should always be informed immediately to the concerned (maintenance) department and the seniors and he will be responsible for getting it repaired. (e.g. computer, telephones, etc.).
6. Outside telephone calls should not be transferred to certain telephone extensions like OT, high-risk areas, etc. which are mainly to be used as intercoms.
7. All the telephonic messages for the director/MS or the consultant who was not available at that time should be neatly written and sent through to their chambers.
8. Reception staff will make sure that the house keeping staff has done their job properly in the area close to the reception.
9. It shall be the duty of the reception staff to prepare a daily report about the admissions, discharges, and transfers on the provided proforma.
10. A logbook (complaint-cum-message book) should be maintained at the reception and the receptionist should read it before starting the shift.
11. As soon as the patient is admitted, (if there is no separate admitting office, or at nights) it should be immediately informed to the concerned ward in-charge, and the consultant in-charge after completion of all formalities of admission.
12. If the patient is referred by an outside consultant, the reference slip details should be entered in the register especially maintained for such record purposes.
13. The details of a patient's bill should not be disclosed to any outsider.
14. For the convenience of the visitors and the patients, PCO facility is provided in the hospital and outside calls are not permitted from the hospital telephones. However, admitted patients can avail the phone facility for inward and outward calls. If any admitted patient makes an outside call, it should be informed to the nurse in-charge of that patient so that an entry can be made in the file.
15. In case of an emergency or casualty, the patient or her/his relatives can use the hospital telephone facility. The same rule applies to PCO if it is out of order. Every outside call shall be charged as per hospital charge schedule.
16. The staff managing these services should always remember that all the ill persons or otherwise may not be literate enough to read English/ Hindi signage, nurse should help such persons.

LINEN KEEPER/HOUSE KEEPING DEPARTMENT IN-CHARGE

The following are the duties of the linen-keeper:

1. To arrange for the supply of the clean linen to all the wards, operation theatre and the OPDs. For this, he will fix a time of linen exchange in consultation with hospital authorities. While making issue, he will check the items for its buttons and drawstrings.
2. Items requiring repair or damaged beyond repair should be kept separately and should be issued.
3. To get the soiled linen from the wards (himself or through housekeeping staff), operation theatre, Wards and the OPDs to replace it with the clean linen.
4. To arrange for the washing of the soiled line from the laundry.
5. Fully responsible for the control of the laundry department.
6. To ensure that the equipment and the machinery of the laundry department are in good state of working at all the times.
7. Ensure that the laundry gets the required material for cleaning the linen (in case it is not outsourced).
8. To count the number of clothes before giving to and taking from the laundry.
9. All clothes received from the laundry, which are not washed up to the mark will be returned to the laundry for rewash, free of cost.
10. To indent for the replacement of the old and worn out linen.
11. To mark the linen with the signage of the hospital so that the hospital linen cannot be mixed with the private linen.
12. He will not allow any unauthorized person to enter the stores.
13. He will keep a ledger to all linen in the store and line issued to various departments. He will make entry for all the items received and issued to various departments.
14. He will check physically the inventory or other departments once in three months.
15. He will also carry out physical verification of his own stock once in 3 months.
16. In addition to these duties, he should also perform all those duties as are assigned to him by his seniors from time to time.

BILLING STAFF (IP)

1. If the billing procedure is computerized the billing supervisor and staff should check the working of all computers.

2. He should check the daily report of admissions, transfers and discharges.
3. He should make daily entries in the patient records regarding the charges for various services provided to the patient.
4. He should check the pending payments from the patients every day and report should be sent to the administrator and ward in-charge to inform to the patient.
5. He should also check the payments made by the patient/attendant and the amounts are properly entered in the patient individual records.
6. He should take the minimum time to prepare a final bill for patient who are getting discharged as per the schedule.
7. One more person should verify the final bill before handing it over to the patient for payment.
8. He should verify the charges for OT and drugs used in OT for patients who have undergone surgical procedure in OT.
9. He should verify all charges mentioned in the case-sheet regarding the procedures like ventilator charges, bed side investigations, monitor, oxygen, etc. and professional fees for consultants.
10. After raising a final bill the case-sheet should be sent to MRD for proper filing.
11. The final bill should be sent to the patient or handover the bill to the attendant at the billing counter for payment.
12. If the bill amount is huge in case of company patients, it should be informed to the concern company medical officer for further sanction of limit.
13. He should send a weekly bill statements to the patients to enable them to pay an advance payment to the hospital.
14. He should coordinate with various departments and TPA help desk for collecting information regarding patient charges and other particulars.
15. He should answer the queries made by the patients/attendants, corporate companies and insurance companies.
16. He should attend the training program conducted by the management.
17. He should help the management in minimizing the discharge procedure by coordinating with various departments and by adopting various methods.
18. He should inform to the computer personnel if there is any breakdown of computers and see that it will be rectified immediately.
19. He should develop a system of making manual bill in case of computer failure.
20. Any other duties assigned by the management.

SANITARY TECHNICIAN

Most of the hospitals up to a capacity of 250 beds do not have such post. Though, it is advisable to recruit one, if the hospital budget allows.

The sanitary technician is responsible for the supervision of the general sanitation of hospital and its surroundings and for implementation of measures necessary to ensure the health of patients and staff.

His duties will cover cleaning of the premises, disposal of waste (including bio-medical waste) as per government norms:

1. All the staff of this department will be under direct control of sanitary inspector, even if they are on contract.
2. He will ensure that all the policies of this department are followed in letter and spirit.
3. To take antirodent and anti-flies measures.
4. He will also ensure safe drinking water is available to hospital patients and staff.
5. He will be responsible (directly or indirectly), for disinfection and fumigation of room after discharge of an infected patient or death. Similarly, he will also supervise the disinfection of non-disposable linen material of that room.
6. If the department is functioning under hospital control, he will maintain an inventory of all consumables and nonconsumable items.

SWEEPERS

They are the most important staff in a hospital. The works they carry are most important for the well being of patients. They should not be neglected and should be handled in a polite manner.

1. Sweeper in the ward/department will be responsible to the sister/nurse in-charge of that area for the general sanitation of that area and helping the nurse in giving bedpans and urinal pots to the patient.
2. In area, which is not under control of the nursing staff, they will be responsible to the person in-charge of such area.
3. Their duties include all that is required to follow all the policies and procedures listed above.
4. They will mop the ward/patient rooms' floors and clean the toilets and sanitary fittings therein.
5. Their duties include washing and disinfecting bedpans and urinal pots.
6. The waste disposal will be as per local government norms.
7. Any other duty assigned by their superiors including nurses of that area.

AMBULANCE DRIVER

1. The driver of an ambulance should hold a license as per the available vehicle (Light motor vehicle license for smaller ambulances and Heavy motor-commercial driving license).
2. He should be an expert in driving a vehicle safety at faster than normal speed.
3. He should be literate and should be trained in handling stretcher and some basic ambulance equipments and should also know a little bit of mechanics.
4. It will be the duty of the driver to keep the vehicle neat and clean and in running condition always.
5. The medical supplies will be checked on daily basis irrespective of the vehicle movements and any loss, damage, consumption will be reported to the in-charge immediately.
6. The supplies will be replenished on urgent basis and details can be inquired of latter about unexplained loss, damage or consumption.
7. The driver of the ambulance will maintain a logbook, which will be checked and signed by the MS/MD on daily basis.
8. In normal circumstances only specified driver will drive the ambulance.
9. Any other person will drive the ambulance in case of emergency only on specific orders by the concerned authorities.

AMBULANCE PARAMEDICAL STAFF

1. We in India put any body-driver, ward boy and nurse or even a doctor who is not properly trained in handling emergencies during transportation.
2. The ambulance paramedics or doctor should be specially trained by ICU in-charge, usually an anesthetist in handling emergencies during the course of transportation. It is always good to impart some training to the ambulance paramedic (also to driver) in handling such situation.
3. He should always check the inventory of medical supplies as per list on every morning.
4. He should minimize his exposure to blood or other body fluids by using suitable gloves, etc.
5. Masks should also be used by ambulance personnel.

CSSD TECHNICIANS

1. The in-charge (supervisor) of CSSD will make sure that he has got an initial stock of recognized sets with him in sufficient quantity.

2. He will be responsible for proper handling of these equipments by him and by staff posted under him.
3. Any breakdown or routine maintenance work has to be carried out on urgent basis. It will be the duty of the supervisor to see that the machines are maintained and are repaired by engineers at the earliest.
4. Proper keeping of the records (inventory) of all fixed assets and instruments in good condition is also a duty of this supervisor.
5. He will do the 'physical checking' of the inventory from the register by himself every month and once in three months by the person posted by the administrator.
6. He will ensure that all the departments getting regular supply from CSSD on regular basis are not put to inconvenience because of any insufficiency on the part of CSSD.
7. He will make sure that only demineralized water is used in sterilizers.
8. Water chambers to generate steam of these sterilizers (if not fed by central steam) are cleaned periodically.
9. He will be totally responsible for maintenance of sterility and hygiene of 'sterile area' in particular and complete area in general.
10. He will be responsible for allocating work to his juniors. All leaves required by CSSD employees should have forwarding and recommending note from the supervisor.

WARD ASSISTANTS AND AYAHS

In hospitals, a new tread is emerging to outsource this requirement. It outsourced the agreement with the contractor should incorporate specific points to cover their duties and responsibilities. Ultimately, they are responsible to the hospital.

They will be responsible to the sister/staff nurses of the ward/department for the performance of duties allotted to them. Their duties will be as follow:

Sometimes, this staffs is hired through contractors. In that case also these staff will directly report to the Nurses. They will report for duty every day to the area nurse.

1. They all will enter the hospital from an entrance marked as "staff entrance".
2. Dusting and cleaning of beds, doors, windows, furniture and fittings, utensils, crockery and cutlery in all rooms of ward/department.
3. Supervision of periodical washing of floors/walls and fittings.
4. Making beds of ambulatory patients and vacant beds as per directions of the area nurse.

5. Transporting patients on stretchers, trolleys or wheel chairs or accompanying them to other departments for investigative, operative procedures.
6. Assistance to medical and nursing staff in the care and treatment of patients.
7. Assistance at handling over linen (soiled or otherwise) and clothing and collection of clean ones in exchange.
8. Errands to departments as required.
9. Medical wastage removing.
10. Any other duty that may be assigned by the superiors.

MALE NURSING ASSISTANT

1. To give bed pan
2. Patient shifting
3. To given patients sponge bath
4. To give patient sitz bath
5. Diaper changing
6. To assist for giving enema whenever required
7. Suction cleaning
8. To assist for dressing the wounds, and other dressings as advised by doctor
9. To assist for preparing patient for surgery
10. To feed food to the patient if necessary
11. Provide assistance to all staff in the performing their duties as and when required
12. To carryout messenger services and when required by the ward staff
13. To maintain co-ordination amongst the co-staff
14. The job holder is required to maintain cleanliness/hygine in and around the hospital premises.

PUBLIC RELATION OFFICERS

The first and foremost duty of the public relation officers (PRO) in a hospital is to help and guide the patients properly in the hospital. The important duties and responsibilities of the public relation officer is:

1. He/she has to make regular rounds in the wards to find out/to get feedback from the patients.
2. He/she has to coordinate with the management staff for rectifying any faults regarding the engineering services like electrical, plumbing, carpentry, etc.

3. He/she should attend on grievances of patients and any issues beyond her/his capacity it should brought to the notice of administrator.
4. He/she should be polite in dealing with the patients and their attendants.
5. He/she should also coordinate with the doctors; any issue relating to the treatment should be brought to the notice of treating doctor.
6. He/she should make sure that the wards are kept clean through the coordination with the ward assistants and ayahs.
7. He/she should maintain the staff movement register in ward to know the staff movements.
8. He/she should educate the patients regarding their rights and responsibilities.
9. He/she should intimate the cost of estimation to the patients.
10. To see that the case-sheets of the discharged patients are sent to MRD department.
11. To remain the patients about their outstanding payments.
12. To monitor the grooming of ayahs and boys.
13. He/she should help code blue, pink, red and brown teams whenever required.
14. He/she will make sure that the signboards are kept properly in the premises by the hospital.

MAINTENANCE SUPERVISOR/FACILITY MANAGER

Maintenance supervision or facility manager is one who supervises the maintenance of entire hospital. He will control the staff working in engineering departments like electricity, plumbing, painting, carpentry, air-conditioning, watch and ward, sweepers and civil department (if any). The maintenance supervisor or facility manager has an important role in day-to-day administration.

- Maintenance of all records regarding the complaints of day today general maintenance of hospital and rectified reports
- He is responsible to keep all license and permission of local authorities and government bodies which are applicable for hospital
- He should monitor the work of maintenance staff
- He should keep the premises clean through his team of Maintenance staff
- He should coordinate with ward and other department staff in case of any fire, or disaster in the premises of the hospital
- He should report the accidents/incidents that occurred during the month to the safety committee for discussion and carryout the rectification measures

- He should supervise the services of security personnel
- Proper care should be taken with regards to the staff, patients, and visitors while civil construction is going in the premises of the hospital
- He should periodically check the electrical, plumbing, air-condition and other engineering equipments to make sure that they are in working condition
- He should help the management to get building permission from local authorities like municipalities, corporation, etc.
- He should also monitor the renewal of licenses, if any, on due dates
- He will make sure that the biomedical wastage is properly handled and disposal according to the pollution control board norms
- He should monitor the sewerage water treatment plant and attend on pollution control board officials where they come for inspection
- Any other duties regarding the maintenance and facility management assigned by the management.

PHYSIOTHERAPIST

He should run the department efficiently under the guidance of orthopedic surgeon, neurologist, cardiologist and other consultants. He should ensure proper privacy and comfort of each patient:

- Proper earthling should be provided for physiotherapy equipments and care should be take while treating a patient as they are electrical equipments
- He should maintain appointment timings given to the patients and reduce the waiting period
- He should prepare roster for the staff working in his department
- He should maintain discipline in the ward
- He should keep the department clean
- He should observe the behavior of the staff especially while delaying with lady patients
- He should make proper arrangements to attend on both outpatients and inpatients in the ward regularly and without delay from the scheduled time
- He should attend on emergency cases
- He should make sure that all the equipments in his department are in working condition
- He should maintain the inventory of the consumables and the equipments.
- If calliberation is required for any equipment it should be done by the authorized and qualified person and keep the certificate in the department
- He should give training to his junior staff and he himself should attend training program conducted by the management.

CHAPTER 29

Sensitive Issues in Hospitals: Role of Administration

Generally in any hospital Patients faces many problems due to language and Finance problems in addition to their mental depression due the patient condition. Due to mishappenings, misbehavior and mishandling of patients in some hospitals, Patients have their own apprehensions about hospitals. Sometimes, the rules and the procedures of the hospital may irritate the patients and their relatives. The administration also faces many problems in its day-to-day running of the hospital as it has to follow the rules and regulations of the State and the Medical Council of India. In addition to that the law of the land also should be followed by the hospital organizations. The administration has to play an important role to overcome these issues. Though the object of the hospital is to generate more money to run the hospital effectively, it should also emphasize and cultivate the culture of service to the patients among the healthcare workers which will boost up the image and the good will of the hospital. Some of the issues of the administration, patients and their relatives are given in this chapter.

BROUGHT IN DEAD CASES

In case of road accident or massive heart attack patients may be brought by an ambulance, auto or by a car to the hospital for treatment. Those patients should be received at the casualty medical officer (CMO) and she/he should check the vital parameters and do the initial assessment. Sometimes, the patients may die during the transit itself but the attendants may not be aware of it. They come to the hospital, then in the casualty medical officer will declare that the patient was brought dead. Since it is a medicolegal case the CMO has to inform the police in a prescribed format. Sometimes, the patient attendants are not willing to handover the body to police. In such a situation, 'death certificate' becomes an issue. But the CMO can issue the death certificate after checking the vital parameters and the reason for death in the certificate will be mentioned as 'brought dead'. In such situations, he should handover the body to police officer of the nearest police station for investigations (postmortem). If the casualty medical officer does not report to the police he is responsible to the court of law in case of any dispute arises. This sensitive situation can be handled by the medical officer and senior nursing officer of casualty by counseling the patient's relatives by explaining the facts of medical law.

REPLACEMENT OF DRUGS

When the patient is brought to the casualty in a critically ill condition he/she may be taken into emergency ward or ICU ward. Here the doctors on duty provide an emergency treatment to the patient by using the emergency drugs and disposables from the ward stock. Once the patient's condition is stabilized, the ward in-charge nurse will ask the patient attendant to replace the drugs and disposables used for the patient. But the problem arises when the patient could not be saved in spite of sincere efforts made by the doctors. The normal procedure in any hospital is that the doctor will declare the death of a patient and inform the relatives about the time of death. Later the ward in-charge nurse may ask the attendant to replace the drugs and disposables used on patients when he was in a serious condition before her/his death. But the relatives of the dead person may get annoyed and blame the hospital for collecting money for the medicine used for the dead person in ICU or casualty by mistaking the reason for replacement of drugs. To avoid such situation, it is suggested to charge the cost of drugs and disposables used on patients (before his death) in the final bill under the head 'Drugs used in the ward' and replace those items for inventory purpose in the wards by sending a separate indent to pharmacy.

REFUSAL FOR ADMISSION

The casualty in any hospital is a place where all the patients are admitted for inpatient treatment either for chronic disease or for emergency treatment who comes directly to the hospital with/without any reference. After initial assessment in the 'casualty ward', the CMO transfers the patient either to ICU or to the wards depending upon the patient condition. Sometimes, the patients can be refused to receive by CMO for admission on the following grounds:

a. Nonavailability of beds in casualty or ICU for sick patients.
b. Nonavailability of life supporting equipment like ventilators.
c. Nonavailability of specialty wards like burns ward, isolated ward, etc.

Since a patients relatives approaches a hospital due to his/her belief in the treatment offered there, they may not like to be refused admission. In that situation if casualty medical officer informs the patient or attendant that he can not admit patient's for the above mentioned reasons, they will become violent. It would be difficult task for CMO to convince the patient or his attendant. Such a delicate situation can be over come by tactically handling patients by CMO. He can explain to the patients or relatives that it is not intentional and also the consequences of delay in treatment.

TERMINAL PATIENTS

Sometimes, the ventilator patient becomes critically ill and treating doctors in ICU may feel that the chances for survival is very less. In such situation some of the patients' attendants ask to discontinue the treatment due to financial constraints. Since the removal of the ventilator may lead to death in the hospital premises, the attendants may ask for 'death certificate'. The best way to deal with the situation is to, discharge patient on request of patient attendant following the procedure for 'discharge against medical advise'. The patient should be shifted to his home or to the other hospital with an Ambu bag. In addition to obtaining duly signed consent form for refusal of treatment, the nearest relative like wife/husband/mother/father/son/daughter, etc. should give a handwritten letter in any language stating that he/she is willing to take the patient who is on ventilator against medical advice and management is not responsible for any consequences. Legal opinion can be obtained in such cases and the same should be documented.

REDO TESTS

When the patient has been asked to take the test once again due to non co-operation of patients she/he will accept for the same. But if the patient has been asked to repeat the test by a doctor or a ward nurse due to the negligence of hospital staff like loss of blood sample, loss of reports, loss of X-ray film, due to lysen of blood, etc. the patient or patient's attendant, especially in case of a child will create an unpleasant situation in the department. Such sensitive situation needs to be handled diplomatically and the staff should care at most care such situations.

OUTPATIENT DEPARTMENT

The secretary of OP receptionist gives appointment to patients in order to avoid long waiting by the patients. Usually patients come early with a wish to meet doctor prior to their appointment time. This will lead to crowd in OP area. Sometime, the doctors may not be able to come due to emergency situation, or due to personal reasons. Waiting by patient in OP department can be avoided by properly calculating the time the consultant doctor takes for each patient. If a consultant takes 15 minutes. for each patient, 5 patients can be asked to come in the first hour. So that in case one patient fails to turn up, doctor's time is not wasted. The consultant should also inform the receptionist if any change in her/his schedule, which must be informed to the patients over the phone by the receptionist. Hence, proper communication at various levels ensures smooth co-ordination and better patient care in OP department.

RECEPTION

The main reception in any hospital is the area where the prime details of patients are entered into the patient records of the hospital. The general procedure of admission of any patient in the hospital is that, the patient attendant, if the patient is sick or the patient himself will go to the main Reception and submit the personal details like name, age, address, spouse or parent's name, etc. Though 90% of the patients give their details correctly, some of the patients or their attendants submit the wrong details in a hurried manner or due to ignorance. Sometimes, the receptionist may also enter wrong particulars in the computer or in the registers. At the time of discharge or in case of death of a patient these wrong particulars of patients, i.e. wrong spelling of name, initial, age and address will badly reflect in discharge summary or in death certificates. It would be difficult to alter or change these particulars once they are entered into the computer at the time of discharge or after discharge as all the bills and forms in the case-sheet are filled with the particulars given at the time of admission.

As there are number of types of patients like cash paid patients, company patients, cashless treatment patients, staff, etc. the type of patient should be entered on the case-sheet for easy reference by the nursing staff and billing staff. Fail to enter the type of the patient in the case-sheet may lead to wrong billing and delay in the preparation of the final bill.

The patients are allotted beds in a hospital based on their condition and the choice of the patient. Hence, the patient's are transferred from bed to bed, either from ICU to the ward, vice versa or general ward to the private room. The transfers of patients within the hospital should be entered correctly in the computer when the transfer takes place, failing which the information about the patient's room is not known and since the bed charges differs, it will affect the billing too.

The patients referred by the public sector undertakings or insurance companies are eligible for particular types of room. It is mentioned in their reference letters. If the eligibility of the room is not mentioned, the patient can be admitted in any category of room as per the choice of the patient. In case of eligibility, the patients should be admitted in particular room according to their eligibility. If patient selects a higher category of room she/he has to pay the difference of room rent separately at the time of discharge. Sometimes, the hospital will admit these patients in a higher category of room due to non-availability of the eligible room. In such cases the patients will refuse to pay the difference of amount and the company may or may not pay the difference of room rent. To avoid such situation the ward in-charge can take a prior consent from the patient for payment of difference of bed charges.

Generally there is an exception when the patient is in ICU or in emergency ward where the bed charges are higher than the eligibility room.

SUGGESTIONS/COUNTER MEASURES

The main reception is a front office of the hospital and the goodwill and the image of the hospital depends on the behavior and the attitude of the persons working in reception. It is also an entry point for all the particulars of the patient for all his future records, hence the receptionist should be selected carefully by the management. Persons with good communication skills, pleasant behavior, helping nature, are usually placed in the reception. All the receptionists should be given training on maintenance of records, the public speaking and in communication skills.

The patient or their attendants should be asked to fill the preprinted forms with the correct details of the patients or a computer can be provided for them to enter the particulars of the patient which will be transferred to the main reception computer. In the case of illiterate patients the receptionist can help them in entering the particulars. The receptionist should take much care in entering the bed transfers and also other particulars in the case-sheet.

BILLING

In administrative departments billing is one of the most important department. The entire revenue of the hospital depends on the billing department. Loss of revenue to the hospital can be avoided by proper entry of the charges by the billing staff. The charges for various procedures done, investigation charges, bed charges etc. should be collected from various departments for billing to the patients. Hence the billing staff should have a good rapport and coordination with the other staff.

Common issues in billing department are:

1. Delay in billing procedure.
2. Problems arising due to noncoordination between ward and billing section.
3. Wrong entries in bill.
4. Wrong calculation of charges.
5. Lack of politeness among staff.
6. Problems arising due to noncoordination between billing staff and TPA help desk.
7. Delay in getting charges from OT and professional fees from doctors.
8. Final bill amount exceeding the estimated amount from patient's view.
9. Break down of computers.
10. Allotment of beds with higher bed charges than the eligibility of patients in case of company or insurance patient.
11. Collection of outstanding payments from the patients.

The first and common complaint about the billing procedure is delay in getting final bill from the billing department. The patient expects the final bill as soon as the doctor advises for discharge. Though the hospital information system is developed on local area network (LAN), some of the charges to be entered manually by seeing the case sheet like drugs used in the ward, test done in the ward, ventilation charges, monitor charges, procedures done in the ward, etc. Generally when the doctors go for rounds in the morning or evening, he will decide about the discharge of a particular patient based on his health condition. He immediately tells the patient or attendant that the patient can go home at any time and is fit for discharge. Then the case-sheet is sent from the ward to the billing section which will take time as the nursing officer will also be in rounds along with the doctors briefing about the patients in her ward. By that time the doctor completes his rounds in a ward having 12 beds it would have taken minimum of 60 minutes if he takes 5 minutes for the examination of each patient.

The nursing officer can send a case sheet of a patient who is getting discharged only after entering all the details and charges. In this process, there will be delay in raising the final bill. The patient expects the bill to be ready in the billing counter as soon as he goes there for bill settlement. There is also a chance for the billing clerk to commit mistake in calculating charges or making entries in the bill, etc. due to pressure in the counter.

SUGGESTIONS FOR QUICKENING THE BILLING PROCESS

The first way to minimize the delay is by providing computers in the ward apart from the investigation departments and operation theatres. The charges pertaining to each patient should be entered in the computer in daily basis by the nursing officer or ward in-charge or floor supervisor, etc. If the hospital cannot afford to invest so much of money on computers, the system of sending daily charge statement of all patients to the billing section should be developed.

Secondly, the maximum time taken to raise the final bill should be displayed in front of the billing counter. The ward nurse should also inform to the patient the approximate time to get the final bill. Prior information to the customer about the discharge procedures will always help the management.

ESTIMATED COST OF TREATMENT

One of the patient rights is to get estimated cost of treatment. As a part of fulfilling the right of patients, hospitals should give an estimated cost of treatment for which the patient is admitted. But sometimes, the hospital bill exceeds the estimated cost.The patient or attendant will get upset after receiving the final bill. The increased cost may be due to postoperative complications, the number of days stay, change in line of treatment, usage of costly drugs, etc. It would be difficult for patients/ attendants to make arrangements for funds to settle the hospital bills if they asked to pay huge amounts without prior intimation about the outstanding bill amount.

SUGGESTIONS

Hence, it is suggested to inform the patient's attendant the estimated cost of treatment based on the primary diagnosis and also should be informed that the cost may differ if the line of treatment changes due to further prognosis. It is always better to take signature of the patient/attendant in the prescribed form that he was informed about the estimated cost of treatment. In any case if the actual cost of treatment exceeds the estimated cost, the nursing officer or RMO should inform again the patient/attendant the extra cost of treatment by giving the reason for the same. It should also be mentioned in the case-sheet and should have got an acknowledgement by the patient or attendant.

EFFECTIVE FUNCTIONING OF BILLING SECTION

- If the billing procedure is computerized the billing supervisor and staff should check the working of all computers
- He should check the daily report of admissions, transfers and discharges
- He should make daily entries in the patient records regarding the charges for various services provided to the patient
- He should check the pending payments from the patients everyday and report should be sent to the administrator and ward in-charge to inform to the patient
- He should also check the payments made by the patient/attendant and the amounts are properly entered in the patient's individual records
- He should take the minimum time to prepare a final bill for patient
- The final bill should be double checked before handing it over to the patient for payment
- He should verify the charges for OT and drugs used in OT for patients who have undergone surgical procedure in OT
- He should verify all charges mentioned in the case-sheet regarding the procedures like ventilator charges, bed side investigations, monitor, oxygen, etc and professional fees for consultants
- The final bill should be sent to the patient or handover the bill to the attendant at the Billing counter for payment
- If the bill amount is huge in case of company patients, it should be informed to the concerned company medical officer for further sanction of limit
- He should send a weekly bill statement to the patients to enable them to pay an advance payment to the hospital
- He should coordinate with various departments and TPA help desk for collecting information regarding patient charges and other particulars
- He should answer the queries made by the patients/attendants, corporate companies and insurance companies
- He should attend the training program conducted by the management
- He should help the management in minimizing the discharge procedure by coordinating with various departments and by adopting various methods

- He should inform to the computer personnel if there is any breakdown of computers and see that it will be rectified immediately
- He should develop a system of making manual bill in case of computer failure.

PHARMACY

Some of the common complaints about pharmacy are:

NONAVAILABILITY OF DRUGS

One of the major complaints from the patients in the hospitals is Non-availability of medicines prescribed by the consultants. It is the duty of top management to see that the medicines prescribed by the consultants regularly are kept in the pharmacy. The nonavailability of medicines may create the panic situation among the patients as the medicines cannot be given to the patients in right time and also it may cause loss to the management.

Every hospital should have a drug formulary. It should contain all the medicines available in hospital pharmacy. The pharmacy in-charge should have a system of procuring these drugs from the distributor and dealers or from the market on time and his responsibility is to see that the drugs mentioned in the drug formulary are available in pharmacy. Pharmacy should function round the clock. Before prescribing a new drug for a patient by the consultant it should be approved in pharmacotherapeutic committee. All new drugs approved based on requirement by the committee shall be included in the drug formulary and stock should be kept in the pharmacy.

DELAY IN ISSUING MEDICINES

The busy hours in pharmacy are during 9 am to 12 noon and 4 pm to 7 pm. Most of the consultants are on rounds during these timings and prescribe medicines for patients. Similarly the outpatients will be more during these timings. Due to the heavy crowd in the pharmacy during the morning and evening timings the issue of medicines to the patients will take long time. Especially the patients who wanted to buy a less number of medicines like 2 or 3 drugs has to wait for a long time if the crowd is more If the billing department and the issue departments are functioning both for outpatients and inpatients in pharmacy, it will cause delay in issuing medicines to both outpatients and inpatients.

In case of emergencies the patient's attendants will become restless to stand in a queue for billing as well as for collecting medicines from the counter. The general complaint in any hospital regarding the pharmacy is delay in the supply of medicines and waiting time is more.

To avoid overcrowding in pharmacy the management can have a system of supplying medicines to inpatients directly by the hospital staff as per the advice of the doctors and also have separate counter for less number of medicines and out patient's sales.

HOSPITAL-ACQUIRED INFECTION

It is a fact that some people checking into the hospital face risks. Expecting to get better, some actually wind up getting worse.

We have all heard the horror stories about hospital risks after surgery. There is the danger of medical complications, like bleeding or infection. Then there are the human errors, like getting the wrong drug or dosage. "Even though the hospital got a lot of well-trained people working very hard, they are still people,"says Fran Griffin, Director in Camebridge University. And people sometimes make mistakes. Another top hospital risk is infection with bacteria or virus. Hospitals are loaded with nasty bugs. According to the CDC, there are 1.7 million healthcare-associated infections every year; 22% are infections of surgical wounds. Even more 32% are urinary tract infections. The rest are infections of the lungs, blood, and other parts of the body.

MEDICATION ERRORS

"Far and away, the most serious hospital risk is a medication error," says Carolyn Clancy Director for AHRQ, Rock Ville.

- Wrong medicine
- Wrong dose
- Wrong time
- Wrong patient.

A 2006 report from the Institute of Medicine estimated that every year, there are 450,000 injuries resulting from medication errors in hospitals, and perhaps many more that are unreported. What is especially frightening about these hospital risks is they seem completely beyond control. How can stop a doctor's poor handwriting on a prescription from being misread by a pharmacist or nurse? But there are things that patient can do to reduce this hospital risk. Before surgery, he need to make sure that his doctor, his surgeon, and everyone else involved in his care know about every single medicine—whether prescription, over-the-counter, or herbal supplement—that he uses. To make it easier, can just put all of his medicines in a bag and bring them to the hospital.

METHICILLIN RESISTANT *STAPHYLOCOCCUS AUREUS* (MRSA)

One of the most frightening hospital infections that can pick up is methicillin-resistant *Staphylococcus aureus* (MRSA)—a type of staph infection that's resistant to many antibiotics. A 2007 study by the Association for Professionals in Infection Control and Epidemiology (APIC) suggested that almost one out of every 20 hospital patients is either infected with MRSA or carries it.

"The risk of MRSA is growing," and. "It's getting more common and more resistant to antibiotics."says Clancy.

The best way to prevent this infection is by giving correct antibiotics before and after surgery. Then after surgery, the best protection is not allow anyone including doctors and nurses to touch the patient without washing their hands.

PNEUMONIA

Although some might think of pneumonia as a minor complication, it can be quite serious. After urinary tract infections and wound infections, it is the most common hospital acquired infection.

According to the CDC, estimates of hospital pneumonia's mortality rate are as high as 33%. It is most common in people who are in the intensive care unit or on ventilators. This will also be called as ventilator-associated pneumonia (VAP).

Pneumonia is a common hospital risk after surgery for several reasons. During recovery, one might naturally take shallow breaths, since she/he is on his back and breathing deeply may be painful. After surgery, many people also have a partial collapse of the lung tissue called atelectasis, which further weakens lung function. All of this can make it easier for bugs that cause pneumonia to gain a foothold.

So, it is recommended that the patients should try to take 10–15 big breaths every hour to avoid this hospital risk, according to Angood. If patient is a smoker, she/he should quit smoking or at least stop for a week or two before surgery. Just a short break can make a big difference in the health of patient's lungs. Aspiration pneumonia has a more specific cause. It develops when patient breathe in fluids, like vomit. This can happen after anesthesia because his normal coughing reflexes may be suppressed. The best way to avoid this type of pneumonia is to follow doctor's advice about not eating or drinking after midnight the day before surgery. If he does not have anything in his stomach to vomit up, the danger of aspiration pneumonia is quite low.

DEEP VEIN THROMBOSIS (DVT)

"DVT, it clearly ranks as one of the more significant risks after surgery," says Clancy.

DVT—or deep vein thrombosis—is the development of a blood clot, typically deep in the veins of the leg. If the clot breaks free and travels through the bloodstream, it can get lodged in the arteries of the lungs, cutting off the blood supply of oxygen. This complication, called a pulmonary embolism, can be fatal.

Surgery significantly increases the risks of DVT for several reasons. If the patient is immobile in bed, his circulation gets worse. That makes the blood more likely to pool and clot in his legs. Also the blood vessels in his legs can become very "relaxed" during the anesthesia used for surgery and the blood can slow down its movement enough to form a clot, especially if the vessel has prior damage (for example, by way of a previous history of a broken leg) . The trauma of surgery itself also increases the blood's clotting tendency. Without preventive treatment, the odds of getting DVT after a prolonged major surgery are 25%. For some surgeries, like joint replacement, the odds of DVT are more than 50%. Fortunately, careful use of blood thinners can slash the risk of DVT without increase in the risk of bleeding.

Another method of DVT prevention is like stretching and as per doctor's advice, getting up and walking, will get patient's blood circulation back to normal.

BLEEDING AFTER SURGERY

While clotting is a risk for DVT, uncontrolled bleeding after surgery causes problems of its own.

However, there is good news "bleeding after surgery is not as much of a problem as it once was".

Griffin says, thanks to improved surgical techniques. Still, you should make an effort to lower the risks further.

That starts with making certain that treating doctor knows every medication —vitamins, supplements—that he use. Common medicines—like the painkillers aspirin and ibuprofen—can thin the patient's blood, increasing the risk of bleeding. The patient has to stop taking any medicine that might have this effect a week or two before surgery. If you forget and take one of these drugs, "There is a simple blood test that can be done to check if your blood is too thin for surgery," says Griffin. "But your doctor might not think to do the test unless you tell him or her."

Also mention if you've ever had excessive bleeding before, even for something minor, like the removal of wisdom teeth. "The biggest predictor of serious bleeding after surgery is history of having bled after surgery before," says Clancy. If your surgeon knows, he or she can take precautions.

ANESTHESIA COMPLICATIONS

While many patients still worry about anesthesia, experts say that it is really quite safe these days.

"There is no doubt that the biggest advances in improving surgical safety have been in anesthesiology," "They have made enormous strides." Although rare, some people have allergies to certain anesthetics. Rare genetic conditions can also trigger anesthesia complications. "It is always worthwhile to check and see if any other family members have had a bad reaction to anesthesia," Clancy says. If Doctor suspect the patient might be at risk, the patient may have testing done before the surgery.

OPERATION THEATERS

Operation Theaters are one of the important high risk areas in the hospital. Multispecialty hospitals are not complete without operation theaters. There should be minimum of two operation theaters in any hospital. The multispecialty hospitals will have separate operation theaters for major specilities like cardiac, neuro, liver transplant, etc.

Some of the common issues are:

1. Waiting time in operation theater
2. Postponement of surgery due to nonavailability of doctors
3. Complications while doing surgery
4. Non recovery of patient from anesthesia after surgery
5. If there is any leftover of gauze or cotton in the abdomen by surgeons by mistake
6. Lack of proper postoperative care
7. Re-do surgery for any reason/complication.

The common problem of surgical patients is waiting for surgical procedure beyond the scheduled time. The treating consultant surgeon will fix the time for surgical procedure based on the severity of the problem. But there will be a delay in taking patient to the operation theater for surgery from the ward for many reasons:

a. Due to delay in preparation of patient.
b. Due to delay in previous surgical procedure.
c. Due to nonavailability of surgeons in time.

d. Due to nonavailability of ward staff to shift the patient.
e. Due to delay in getting investigations done.
f. Due to delay in getting reports from the investigation departments.

The patient and attendant will become restless and sometimes shout at the ward staff as the patient is in starvation, chances of skipping the auspicious time, etc.

The other delicate situation where the patient and the attendant get irritated is the postponement of surgery due to non availability of theater or surgeon. Sometimes the elective surgery will be postponed as some other patient has been already posted in Theatre for surgery as an emergency case, i.e. Head injury, acute appendicitis, brain hemorrhage, etc.

Secondly, the surgery will be postponed as the surgeon is held up in other hospital or he is out of town. The surgery will also be postponed due to noncooperation of the patient or the patient is not fit for surgery due to some infection or other health problems. Under this situation the patient and the attendants will compromise and convince for the postponement of surgery as the hospital and doctor are not responsible for the postponement. While doing surgery suddenly the patient may become sick and the surgery becomes complicated for many reasons. It would be very difficult to convince the patient attendants under this situation as the patient has been taken inside the theatre in a good condition. If the surgical procedure is a complicated one or the patient is very sick and there is no other alternative except the surgical procedure, the treating consultant surgeon should explain the situation to the patient attendants, so that the patient attendants will prepare mentally for the consequences/untoward incidents. Most of the patients are afraid of surgery not because of surgery but for anesthesia. They have their own apprehensions about anesthesia. Whatever may be the reasons may be sometimes the patient's condition will become bad after surgery and they will not recover from the anesthesia. They will be connected to the ventilators. Ultimately, the issue comes to the administration and the management has to face the consumer redress forum. Hence, the hospital should have a very good team of anesthetists who are well experienced and trained to attend any type of surgical procedure with prolonged number of hours.

Secondly, the anesthetist should counsel the patient and the attendant before surgery and explain about the procedure and complications if any.

REEXPLORATION OF SURGERY

Sometime, the patient has to undergo a surgical procedure for second time due to infection or opening of the wound or sutures, etc. Generally in cardiac surgery or abdominal surgery, this re-do surgery takes place. Though this type of re-do surgeries are rare but it cannot be avoided if there is any infection in surgical site or the wound is not healed or the sutures are opened after surgery. No one may be responsible for a redo surgery but the staff in OT, surgical ward and doctor should follow strictly the infection control measures and hand wash techniques at least to minimize redo surgeries.

POSTOPERATIVE CARE

To buy either domestic appliance (electrical) machines, biomedical equipments, one is being particular about after sales service.

Similarly, postoperative care is very much required for surgical patients. Though the surgical procedure is successfully completed, the patient may get an infection and become initially ill after surgery if the postoperative care is not good. Sometimes, it may lead to the death of a patient. Hence the postoperative care is an important as the surgery and the anesthetist, surgeon and other ward staff should take utmost care of patients after surgery. All the issues mentioned above can be solved by convincing patients or attendants and the negligence of duties of staff can be rectified by counseling and training. But the frightening issue is the leftover of foreign bodies inside the body of a patient while doing surgery by mistake and close the skin. Generally no one will open and try to find out how the surgery has been done and whether the surgery was done correctly or not. Based on the symptom and relief from the problem it will be understood that the surgery is successful. Though it is not the intention of a surgeon to leave something inside, but the result will be very complicated and difficult to convince the patient and attendant once it is found or if there is any side effect. It may prompt the patients to go for consumer redress forum for compensation. So, the OT staff and the surgeons should be very careful while doing surgery and the OT Nurse attending the procedures should count and check the instruments, gauze and cotton bundles etc before closing the surgery.

To avoid such complaints, kindly go through the check list mentioned in Chapter 14: operation theaters.

PUBLIC RELATION OFFICER

Since the public relation officer (PRO) is one who interacts with patients every day he/she gets the complaints from the patients. Most of the time a patient may not want to complaint against the doctor or the ward nurse while he is in the ward, taking treatment with the fear that he may be deprived of the proper treatment if he/she complaints. Hence, the patient expresses their real feelings to the public relation officer. This way the PRO will play an important role in attending the grievances of patients and also act as a bridge between the patient and the management. If the PRO is efficient and has the communication skills and is amicable and has a friendly nature, most of the issues or problems in the wards or the departments can be easily solved. The management should take proper care while appointing a PRO with the above mentioned qualities and fix the duties and responsibilities to PRO.

GENERAL ISSUES

One of the general complaints by the patient in multi specialty hospitals is that the specialist spends minimum time with the patients. Generally, the patients and attendants have doubts and also would like to have the clarification regarding the treatment and also the condition of the patient. Any human being is emotional when his kith and kin is sick and admitted in a hospital for treatment. Some of the economically backward patients are ignorant and they do not know what is happening in the hospital and what type of treatment given to the patient. But it is not the same in case of educated patients/attendants. They would like to know each and every procedure and medicines given to the patient. They will have more doubts and points to be clarified by the consultant. They will be waiting for the consultant regular visit so that they can ask the doctor. To their surprise some of the consultants spend less than a minute or two with the patients. They may not give any time for attendants to discuss or interact. Having spending so much of money in the hospital when the patient does not know the line of treatment, condition of the treatment, probable date of discharge, etc. the patients get upset. Still the patients will not complain about the consultant because he is afraid where he will be deprived of the treatment. Secondly, the patient is also in a way confident on the treatment given by the consultant doctor.

LACK OF INFORMATION/COMMUNICATION TO THE PATIENTS

Providing correct information to the patient is one of the important aspects of the management in hospitals. It is also a right of a patient to get correct information regarding the approximate cost of treatment, the number of days required to stay in the hospital, the condition of the patient, the diagnosis details, the chances of recovery if the patient is critically ill, etc. Most of the complaints from the patients regarding the treatment is mainly due to non availability of information. If a patient is informed in advance by the ward in-charge or the resident medical officer about the details mentioned above, most of the problems regarding the treatment can be avoided. In case of the patient not responding to the treatment the attendant should be informed about the progress of the patient and condition of the patient by the resident medical officer or treating consultant. This may avoid unpleasant situations later. The other problem regarding the information is that sometimes the patient/attendant will get information about the condition of patient especially when the patient is in ICU/emergency ward, from the ward boys/ayahs/housekeeping boys. As the patient's attendants will be anxious to know about the condition of their family members who is in ICU will be happy to know whatever the information they get from the lower cadre staff. But, when it differs from the actual fact that patient is sick, they will get disappointed and get a wrong impression about the hospital. Different information from different people will create confusion in the minds of patients/attendants. Hence, the hospital should have strict policies and system of informing the patient/attendant regarding the condition/progress of the patient by authorized doctors only.

ACTUAL COST OF TREATMENT IS NOT KNOWN

It would be very difficult for a patient or an attendant to know the exact amount he is going to spend in the hospital. The hospital bill is mainly dependent on the number of days of stay, the category of bed, the bed charges, disease, cost of medicines, investigations, professional/surgeon's fees, etc. The hospital administration can give an approximate cost of treatment at the time of admission based on illness. There are a lot of differences in actual cost of treatment between hospitals to hospitals. The patient/attendant would have mentally prepared for a certain amount for the treatment in a particular hospital. If the bill amount exceeds his calculations he may find difficult in arranging the funds for settling the hospital bills. Even then he would like to continue with the treatment in the same hospital as it might otherwise highly satisfactory services. Under these circumstances it is difficult to convince the patient/attendant for making payments to the hospital in case of failure of patient to recover. Hence, the management should have a proper system of informing the patient/attendant, the estimate cost of treatment at the time of admission itself. If this amount exceeds due to various reasons, it should also be informed on a daily basis. Taking the signature from the patient or the responsible attendant in a prescribed cost estimation form whenever they are informed about the approximate cost of treatment is a safer method.

LANGUAGE

Most of the multi specialty hospitals in metropolitan cities get patients not only from the city but also get patients from the neighboring states. One of the common barriers for the other state patients is language. They go to the city hospitals for treatment as proper facilities are not available in their home town. Sometimes the patients travel quite distance crossing 2 or 3 States for treatment as the particular specialty is not developed in their home town. When a north Indian patient comes to south India, he will hear a totally different language except English which he may know. But the lower cader of a staff in a hospital may not know English. Since patients from other states do not know the local language they will be under the impression that they are being cheated by the staff. They will also find it difficult to communicate their problems to the staff and in the same manner they cannot understand the instructions given by the staff. To make the patient comfortable the hospital should provide an interpreter who knows the minimum of major languages to communicate and help the other state patients. The hospital can also provide a help desk staffed by people who know many languages to guide patients properly.

FOOD

Food is another problem for outside patients. Mostly north Indians will take chapattis and dhal whereas the south Indians will take rice. If the hospital does not have the facility to serve food for outsiders, the patient attendants have to go outside the hospital for their food. Generally the hospital will provide diet for patients and the attendants staying along with the patient in the room. The hospital canteen will follow certain timings. The patients admitted during night timings will find difficult to get even a cup of milk for patients.

Though the canteen facility is a supporting service in a hospital, diet is as important as medicine for patients. Timely food to patients helps proper medication. Delay in supply food may lead to delay in medication. Some of the hospitals are not permitting patients to bring food from outside as outside food may cause food poisoning to the patients. It is also a difficult task to satisfy all the patients with regard to the quality and taste of the food as each one will have a different taste. In hospitals the diet should be supplied to the patients based on the recommendation of the dieticians and the treating doctor. The hospital can also have a 24 hours service of coffee, milk, bread, etc. for the patients who come for admission during nights.

ATTENDANTS STAY IN THE HOSPITAL

Most of the multispecialty hospitals may not have facilities for attendants of ICU/EMR patients to stay in the premises of the hospital. As it is a policy of the hospitals not to allow attendants to stay along with the patient in critical areas like intensive care unit, emergency wards, casualty, etc. the attendants have to wait outside the ward or sleep under the trees or in hot sun. They feel that they are paying thousands of rupees to the hospital but the hospital is not providing any shelter for them. Another problem that these attendants lack is toilet facility. Though the hospital provides good care to the patients, by not providing basic facilities to the ICU/EMR attendants, it may affect the reputation of the hospital.

NONAVAILABILITY OF BLOOD FOR TRANSFUSION

In most of the surgical patients, bleeding patients, dingo fever patients, etc. blood transfusion is very much required. The doctor might advise the patient suffering from the above diseases, for blood transfusion. Arranging the suitable blood for a patient is a difficult task for the attendant. If the hospital has got a blood bank in the premises it will make the job of the attendant easy. Otherwise, he has to go from pillar to post to get the suitable blood for the patient. Even if blood is available in blood banks run by NGOs the safety of the blood is very important. Though the same group of blood is available the cross matching of the blood should be done before transfusion. In addition to this the donor should not have infectious diseases, previous history of jaundice, etc. The lab has to test the various parameters to confirm about safety of the blood before giving it to patients. Even if the blood bank is available in the premises of the hospital the blood bank should maintain the standards and the particular group of blood should be available at the right time to supply for the patients. If it is a planned surgery the blood can be arranged as per the requirement by advance intimation to the blood bank. In case of emergency if the required blood is not available in the blood bank then the patient will become restless and panic. The other problem is the transportation of blood from blood banks from outside. If proper care, like ice-box to carry the blood, is not taken the blood will get damaged and not fit for transfusion. Sometimes the blood bank will insist on replacement of blood by the patient's relatives or friends. The outside patients will find it difficult to arrange for donors. Hence, it is suggested to have planned surgeries as far as possible and inform the blood bank in advance the requirement of blood to be supplied on the date of surgery. The blood bank should also keep the rare group blood for supplying to the emergency patients. The blood bank should take utmost care in screening and cross matching the blood before supply to the patients for transfusion. One of the important procedures before transfusion is getting the signed consent form by the patient or attendant.

ROLE OF ADMINISTRATION

Apart from the suggestions/counter measures to reduce the grievances of patients in Hospitals the following factors are essential to minimize the grievances and also solve sensitive issues in day today administration of the hospital:

1. Motivation
2. Training
3. Communication
4. Counseling.

MOTIVATION

Definition: 1

Motivation is the driving force by which humans achieve their goals. Motivation is said to be intrinsic or extrinsic.

Definition: 2

Motivation is something that moves the person to action and continues him in the course of action.

Intrinsic motivation refers to motivation that comes from inside an individual rather than from any external or outside rewards such as money or grades.

Meaning: Motivation is the word derived from the word 'motive' which means needs, desires, wants or drives within the individuals.

It is the process of stimulating people to actions to accomplish the goals.

The work related motivators are:

1. Job attributes
2. Remuneration
3. Co-workers
4. Achievements.

Among these motivators achievements stands first then, remuneration, coworkers and job attributes. The management promises a worker that the management will provide a motor cycle, if he collects the outstanding dues from the companies towards the settlement of hospital bills, he will certainly try to achieve his target. Setting targets or goal setting is one of the successful motivators for workers. Goal setting is a secret of success of a person who is successful in his field. In a hospital all the staff should be motivated by setting their goals.

Though the remuneration is one of the important motivators that studies has revealed, there is a difference in motivating people by remuneration according to gender in hospitals. Generally lady staff working in Hospitals in front office, Reception and in other departments is less motivated by remuneration than the coworkers and job attributes. If the coworkers are not cooperative or harassment by the coworkers by any means, the lady staff may leave the job though the remuneration is reasonable. General survey has reveals that in young medical staff, i.e. RMO nursing staff and other paramedical staff have lower job satisfaction. They plan to change job from one hospital to another either for higher remuneration or higher position or for government jobs. Secondly, their job is routine and monotonous. Thirdly they will have more opportunities in bigger hospitals or by going abroad. It has also been observed that there is more job satisfaction in surgical nursing staff and the staff who are above 55 years. Healthcare professionals tend to be motivated more by intrinsic factor. It implies that this should be a target for effective motivation.

EMPLOYEE MOTIVATION TECHNIQUES

Provide Meaningful and Challenging Work

When people feel that the work they are doing is meaningful, make a difference in some way, and provide them with challenge that stretch them (but also mesh with their ability to achieve them), they become internally motivated. Even the most mundane of work can be motivating if the leader helps the team member put into context the value their work brings either to the consumer or to the organization.

Providing challenging work is also intrinsically motivating for people- the vast majority of people want to feel that their potential is being regularly challenged.

Set Clear Targets and Expectations and Measure Performance

People can be all fired up and ready to give of their best, but if they do not know what excellent performance is or do not know when they have performed excellently or don't know what the aim of the game is … you can pretty well shut the gate on motivation. Spelling out specific targets, goals, and expectations for behavior and performance need not be anything complicated…. It just needs to be done and people need to get regular and timely feedback on how they are performing against those goals.

Give Regular, Direct, Supportive Feedback

Feedback, both positive and performance improving, is vital to continuous improvement and done well it motivates and inspires people to continually move toward using more of their potential. Feedback needs to be timely, specific and presented in such a way that the individual is clear about the behaviors or skills they need to modify (or continue using) in order to improve performance.

Design People's Roles So They Can Use Their Strengths

Assigning people to specific tasks and duties that play to their strengths is one of the best employee motivation techniques. Research has show, more than anything, people who are able to make use of their strengths on a regular basis while at work are more likely to work in teams that perform at higher levels.

Enable Input and Choice in How Work Gets Done

Ninety five percent of people (regardless of their walk of life) want to do a good job, feel pride in what they do, have good relationships with their coworkers and feel they are contributing in a meaningful way. In other words, they are set up by their own internal nature to be a high performer. Unfortunately, in many organizations managers turn the majority of their focus toward the 5% of people who are allergic to work and then instigate rules, policies and practices (such as close supervision) to control this and practices (such as close supervision) to control this 5%. As one can imaging all the does is demean, annoy and demotivate the 95% who are motivated to do their best. They are wasting the talent and natural motivation that the overwhelming majority of people bring to the workplace. Provide people with a forum where they can provide their input in to how work is performed. Giving people control over how they perform the work is intensely motivating.

COMMUNICATION

Good communication is one of the important weapon with which one can solve most of the complaints/problems faced by the patients in the hospital. Through good communication one can convey the things in a better way and convince the patients. Creating good communication skills apart from the training and motivation in the staff is one of the important responsibilities of the management. The management has to develop a team with good communication skills who will interact with the patients in day today administration. Most of the problems are arise regarding the treatment is mainly due to the poor communication skills of the staff. The nursing staff should be trained in such a manner that she should inform patients what they are doing before giving either medicines, injections, procedures, etc. the staff should explain to the patients what medicine she is giving and for what the medicine is being given. If there is any prescribed side-effect for any drug the staff nurse should give the test dose to confirm the side effects then only she has to administer the drug on the patient. Whatever the treatment is given, procedures are done, the medicines are given to the patient if the concerned staff informs or communicates to the patient in advance in a pleasant manner and get signatures from the patients or the attendants wherever it is required the management can avoid most of the complaints from the patients. The staff should have good communication skills not only to deal with the patients but also to convey the things that are happening in the ward to the administration. And the downward communication systems should be developed well the in organization for smooth functioning of the hospital and also to reduce the complaints from the patients.

TRAINING

In any manufacturing industry, information technology, healthcare industry, training places an important role. The management will conduct training programs for new employees or already existing employees on a particular subject or continuous training to their employees on day-to-day developments in their particular fields. The training programs in healthcare industry will also help the management to get the quality of service from the medical and the paramedical staff who are involved directly in the patient care/service. The training is required for the staff working in out patient department, main reception, billing, investigation department wards, and in other departments where the staff are dealing with patients/ attendants directly. The training programs will take the persons from ignorance to maturity/knowledgeable levels and also creates awareness among the staff.

One of the first and foremost program that the management should conduct is an induction program. In this program the HR or the personal manager should introduce the new staff to the organization and also brief them about their duties, responsibilities in the organization. They should also be informed about the scope of service in the organization, the objects of the organization, etc. Every employee working in a hospital should know the services available in the hospital and also the services which are not available in the hospital and the policy of the hospital to refer patients outside for the services which are not available in the hospital. The ward nursing staff and other paramedical staff should know the patients rights and responsibilities. In addition to that all the employees should be aware of their rights and responsibilities in the organization. Whenever a new equipment is introduced staff concerned should get a proper training to operate the equipment efficiently and safely both for the machine and for the operator. The front office, the casualty staff and other staff working in the ward should be trained well to know the policies of the hospital with regard to the nonavailability of beds for patients for inpatient treatment.

The staff working in intensive care unit and the casualty should be aware of the admission and discharge criteria for patients to be admitted in ICU. Handling patients in a hospital is an art and it should be done technically to provide better services to the patients. Especially in regard to the pediatric patients and the vulnerable patients. Special training is required for staff nurses and the other paramedical staff in the wards to teach them how to handle these patients as it requires a special skill. The nursing staff and other paramedical staff also need training in administering chemotherapy drugs to the patients. The administration of chemotherapy drugs on cancer patients requires special attention and also guidance from the treating Oncologists. The preparation of the chemotherapy drugs should be done under the laminar flow system.

One of the important programs of the hospital management is the hospital infection control program. As the hospital associated infection is one of the sensitive issues of the administration in hospitals and it requires lot of efforts by the management to reduce these nosocomial infections. One of the measures to reduce this hospital associated infection is training program for nurses, doctors, and other paramedical staff on controlling infection. This training should be continuous and it should be done regularly for new staff as well as the old staff. One of the techniques which should be used to control the hospital infection is a handwash technique. Every staff from ward boy to the doctor who directly deal with the patient should know the hand washing techniques which consist of six steps. All the staff working in the hospital should undergo a training program in fire fighting also in segregation and disposal of biomedical waste and color codes for the various biomedical wastages.

The staff working in high risk areas should be trained with regard to the usage of personal protective equipments (PPE), i.e. mask, cap, gloves, aprons, etc. In addition to the above training programs one of the important area where the staff working in high risk areas (like casualty, ICU, postoperative wards, etc.) are regarding basic life support (BLS), advanced cardiac or critical life support (ACLS) and continuous pulmonary resuscitation (CPR), etc. The resident medical officers, nursing staff and other paramedical staff working in these high risk areas must undergo training in this area. It can help them to bring back the patients from critical condition to the normal condition.

Participants, in the patients' service skills training program will learn to:

- Practice and learn dealing with difficulty patients
- Educate patients and family members on a hospital stay
- Guide patients and family members through check-in and discharge paperwork
- Acknowledge customer concerns
- Effectively handle all complaints
- Be protective rather than reactive
- Show empathy
- Gain cooperation from unhappy customers
- Work effectively with other staff members to deal with patient concerns
- Provide exceptional customer service for patients and all visitors.

COUNSELING

Counseling in different subjects by different persons in the hospital will help the management to reduce the complaints and also to improve the confidence levels among the patients on doctors and the organization. Some of the areas where patients require counseling is:

1. Operation theater.
2. For diet.
3. End of life care.
4. Before going for any costly tests.

5. Before surgery/procedure.
6. Before any radiotherapy or chemotherapy.
7. Before connecting patient to any life supporting equipments.
8. Before shifting patients to emergency ward/ICU from the ward.
9. For dialysis of patients.
10. For female patients in case of abortion.
11. In case of amputation of limbs.
12. For psychiatric patients.

CHAPTER 30

Architectural Overview Towards Healthcare Projects

A visit to the hospital for most people is wrought with anxiety. Hence, the architecture needs to be environment friendly, healing the mind, body and soul. We cannot simply treat it with the callowness of a general building. It has to be designed with sensitivity towards the user. Hospital is an interactive building with a heart. It is a place for healing and dealing with the various health issues human body is subjected to catering to minds in emotional turmoil.

A healthcare project is very complex in the sense of playing with the goals of satisfying all functional facilities, services, environment and ambience. The appropriate importance needs to be meticulously catered while a hospital interior is designed.

While involving with healthcare projects one need to observe:

- Social responsibility
- Moral responsibility
- Climatically responsive
- Environmental friendly
- Soothing ambience
- Functional fulfillment
- Core architectural principles
- Inter connectivity
- Free flow movements.

The ultimate users of hospital space are:

- Patients
- Doctors
- Supporting services staff
- Public

- Patient's attendants
- Not last but the most important 'The client'.

The key inputs required before starting a project.

- Types of hospital – Service oriented charity
  Government hospital
  Private hospital
  Corporate hospital
- Customer segment – Middle class
  Lower middle class
  Higher middle class
- Area of operation – Urban sector
  Semiurban sector
  Rural sector.

KEY POINTS

The three key points which need to blend into each other creating the perfect solution to healthcare architecture:

I. Function
II. Services
III. Environment.

FUNCTION

- Space requirement areas for dept following norms
- Spaces put in right form
- Orientation of spaces
- Climatic response
- Approach and zoning
- Interlink of zones, depth and rooms
- Scope for expansion—zone, dept and rooms, blocks
- Circulation spaces
- Clarity of movements—clear sense of direction and dimensions sensing with minimal signage
- Buffer areas
- Spaces transferring balance—heavy crowd to lightly crowded
- Passing areas, open areas—no traffic congestion.

SERVICES

- Kitchen, dining to food lifts to patients
- Laundry from CSSD to patient link

- Clear rooms and sterile maintenance
- Dirty corridors and waste management
- Sewage and drainage
- Plumbing and water supply
- Oxygen medical gas lines
- Electricity
- Communication system
- Air-conditioning system.

ENVIRONMENT

- Landscape—outdoors and indoors
- Green architecture—environment friendly
- Energy conservation system
- Form flowing into the landscape
- Colour play soothing yet remarkable
- Materials close to nature and maintenance free
- Elevational massing
- Glazing to the greens
- Corridors and relaxing spaces amidst cool spaces.

METHODOLOGY OF THE PROJECT

STAGE I—DESIGN CONCEPT

I. Site analysis
II. Design concept
III. Schematic plans
IV. Preliminary cost estimate
V. Presentation of conceptual design.

STAGE II—DESIGN DEVELOPMENT

I. Finalization of design based on discussion
II. Working drawing, interior details, elevations, sections and 3D views
III. Revise cost estimate if necessary.

STAGE III—DOCUMENTATION

I. Detailed drawings and specfications for construction
II. Final cost estimate.

STAGE IV—DESIGN EXECUTION

I. Coordination with client and contractors
II. Identifying vendor with design specific information.

III. Complete architecture and engineering support for site execution
IV. Periodic site supervision.

FUNCTIONAL FACILITIES

An architect plays a vital role in understanding the basic functions and requirements for a hospital. He needs to focus on the complete interlink between various facilities and also working towards no criss-cross movements.

Functional facilities requirements for a hospital.

ZONING

Basic zoning plan with respect to type of functional facilities and requirements:

- Hospital zone
- Academic zone
- Administration
- Residential zone
- Amenities and supporting services.

GENERAL HOSPITAL

- Main administration block
- All necessary departments, with OPDs
- IPD wards
- Casualty and emergency block
- Blood bank
- Radiodiagnosis
- OBG with labor ward
- Central investigation laboratories
- OT complex
- ICU complex.

SPECIALTY AND MULTISPECIALTY HOSPITAL

- Cardiology
- Cardiothoracic
- Urology
- Neurology
- Neurosurgery
- Pediatric surgery
- Plastic surgery
- Gastroentrology
- Surgical gastroentrology

- Reception, enquiry, waiting lounges, hospital administration and MRD, common facilities
- OP consultation rooms
- IP general wards as per the mci norms with unit wise along the departments
- Paid wards like special rooms with attached toilets and twin shared rooms
- ICU, CCU
- OT complex with preoperative and postoperative beds
- Cath laboratory center
- MRI, CT scan, C-arms, etc.
- Cardiac investigation centre like TMT, echo, etc. with step 1 observation and holding areas
- Neurolaboratory
- Dialysis center.

HOSPITAL BACKUP SERVICE FACILITIES

- Engineering maintenance departments
- Central workshop
- Central store, drug stores, biomedical stores, etc.
- MRD
- Central sterilization department
- Hospital kitchen and staff dinning
- Central laundry
- Central canteen.

COLLEGE BLOCK WITH FACILITIES

College block with facilities in case of teaching hospital

- Department faculty facilities
- Laboratories
- Demonstration rooms
- Seminar hall/library
- Central library
- Auditorium
- Gallery type of class rooms
- Mortuary
- Animal house
- College administration departments.

RESIDENTIAL FACILITIES

- Residential staff quarters
- Hostels for student—male and female

- Interness hostel
- Residential doctors for Jr and Sr
- Residential doctors for Jr and Sr
- Nurses hostel
- Non-teaching staff quarters
- Play area with gymnasium, etc.

DIVISIONWISE SCOPE OF WORK

ARCHITECTURAL DIVISION

- Digital total station survey of land
- Master layout planning with zoning road network
- Building and block designing with working drawings viz floor plans, elevation sections and other details
- Coordinate with structural and other engineering services for implementation in drawings.

Further revisions details

- Site link for execution and supervision
- Interior planning and detailing.

STRUCTURAL AND OTHER ENGINEERING SERVICES

A. Structural department:
  - Column and center line drawing
  - Excavation, footing and column foundation with reinforcement
  - Plinth beam details
  - Roof slabs and beams reinforcement details
  - Lift well, over head tanks, underground sump, staircase, etc.
  - Structural design reports.

B. Electrical department: Detailed drawings, load calculations, SLD, diagrams, lighting diagrams, etc.

C. Plumbing and sanitary: Layout drawing, details and design reports

D. Estimation and quantities:
  - Preparation of BOQ (bill of quotation)
  - Preparation of specifications as per the client's choice and budget
  - Preparation of cost estimation and tender document.

E. Site visits:
  - Periodical site supervision by respective technical division for an average of twice in a month subjected to the site based on the work progress.

F. Biomedical engineering
   - Identifying medical equipments, laboratory equipments, hospital furniture required by department wise
   - Designing medical gases unit for O_2, N_2O, centralized compressed air and vacuum with appropriate manifolds
   - Identifying materials for operation theatre and finalizing modalities for construction
   - Electrical requirements for rooms with medical equipments such as number of sockets required, rating of sockets and their placements. This includes safety aspects of grounding and circuit breakers
   - Adherence to government protocols for designing equipments with hazardous radiation
   - Designing CSSD with steam sterilizers, ethylene oxide sterilizers, ultrasonic cleaners and space planning for sterile corridor
   - Complying for possible NABH accreditation in the future.

G. Air conditioning: (HVAC) Details drawings and technical specifications, BOQ and tender document.

H. Fire fighting: Details drawings and technical specifications: BOQ and tender documents.

I. Road network and storm water: Road network design, culvert, pavements, cable trenches, storm water trenches, technical specifications, BOQ and tender documents.

J. Landscaping consultant: For detailed designing coordination and execution. Optionally, in-house landscape designing could be taken up in association with a horticulturist, technical specifications, BOQ and tender documents.

K. Communication net work system: Technical specifications, BOQ and tender documents.

L. Water treatment plant, STP, technical specifications, BOQ and tender documents.

M. Special interior designs other than the specified items which is covered in the above schedule, technical specifications, BOQ and tender documents, 2D and 3D views. Animation, walkthrough and power point presentation – of entire site exteriors and main specified areas of interiors with audio effects (script should be approved by client).

PROJECT MANAGEMENT DIVISION

- Selection of site, construction technology and profitability calculation for residential, educational, commercial and industrial projects

- Prepare time schedule charts (CPM, PERT, BAR charts)
- Closely monitoring the design drawings and estimates for a project
- Working out labor and cash flow schedule
- Coordination with various consultants and advisors
- Suggesting measures and programs for quality assurance, testing and reporting
- Safety precautions and accident prevention on site
- Completion of contract formalities
- Arbitration procedures and process
- On site technical team to monitor quality of the work.

HINTS FOR ARCHITECTS

- The minimum space required for General bed is 10’ × 8’ in general ward
- The ICU and emergency ward where the equipments are more the minimum space required for patient is 12’ × 8’
- No separate room should be provided in ICU for patient for better monitoring of patients by the doctors and nursing staff
- The window height should be minimum of 3½" to 4" from the floor levels in general wards where patients cots are laid
- Toilets should be provided in clinical laboratory, for patient to give urine, motion for analysis
- Power points in ICU, OT, wards, departments should be provided for life saving equipments in ICU and operation theater
- Separate power line has to be laid and different color switches should be provided for UPS line for identification purpose
- As a special precaution a separate power cable can be provided for OT and it can be connected to the generator. For any major surgeries like cardiac surgery, renal transplantation, etc. the surgery will be conducted on generator power without depending on the regular power supply, through out the surgical procedure for safety of the patient
- Proper provision should be given for central air-conditioning system and central medical gases supply
- Minimum cabling root should be planned for telephones, computers, cable TV, CCTV, etc. to avoid loss of signals due to lengthy cables. We should also avoid hanging cables to prevent short circuits
- While designing OT complex, provision should be given for dual theaters for organ transplantation surgeries
- Minimum of two barriers before the entry to the theatre should be provided
- General wards, non-air conditioner rooms should have good ventilation and air circulation

- While providing glass to the building on road side especially in ICU and OT, double glass should be provided to avoid dust and noise
- Wherever the central air conditioner ducting false ceiling is planned, the roof height should be minimum of 12 feet
- In radiology department the provision should be given for led doors
- The doors should have enough width to take patients inside with wheel chair or stretchers or cot
- The doctors and nurses station should be adjacent to the casualty/ICU/ Emergency ward and they should have a direct entry from their room to attend on emergency patients
- Avoid slope flooring as much as possible or provide antiskid flooring.
- Provide grab bars in ramps and toilets for safety purpose.

CHAPTER 31

Guidelines for NABH Accreditation for Hospitals

1. What is NABH?
2. Who is the governing body?
3. What is accreditation?
4. How to apply for accreditation?
5. Is there any time limit?
6. Validity of accreditation
7. Who are involved in accreditation?
8. Who can apply?
9. Process to be followed
10. Audit
11. Certificate.

DETAILS OF CHAPTERS IN NABH

1. Standards for hospitals
2. Chapters in NABH
3. Systems
4. Documentation
5. Training program
6. Policies
7. Manuals
8. Scope of service and registers to be followed
9. Infection control
10. Safety manuals
11. Key indicators
12. Committees
13. Quality assurance committee

14. Feedback and follow-up
15. Key points.

To start a tea stall or an idly shop one has to get a license from the local authorities. But to start a hospital where patients are treated, No license or permission is required to be obtained from any local bodies except for buildings and sale of medicines.

So far there is no regulatory body for hospitals, quality of treatment and medical standards of the hospitals are not being regulated or monitored by any authority, local body, regulatory body, etc. only the consumer redressal forum is acting on complaints from the patients for any deficiency of services rendered by the hospital doctors, staff, etc.

1. WHAT IS NABH?

The Quality Council of India (QCI) has set up a constituent board called National Accreditation Board for Hospitals and Healthcare Providers (NABH). This Board is to establish and operate accreditation program for healthcare providers.

NABH—National Accreditation Board for Hospitals and Healthcare Providers.

2. NABH BOARD COMPOSITION

i. Chairman
ii. Indian Medical Association
iii. Consumer Coordination Council
iv. Insurance Regulatory and Development Authority
v. Indian Nursing Council
vi. Sri Chitra Thirunal Institution and Medical Science and Technology
vii. Direct general, Armed Forces Medical services
viii. Department of Biotechnology
ix. Post Graduate Education Institution (on basis)
x. CEO NABH (Member Secretary)
xi. Chair, Health Committee
xii. Chair, Health Committee—ASSOCHAM
xiii. Chair, Health Committee—FICCI
xiv. Academy of Hospital Administration (AHA)
xv. Ex-Office Members
    a. Secretary General—QCI
    b. Chair – Accreditation Committee—NABH
    c. Chair – Technical Committee—NABH
    d. Chair – Appeal Committee—NABH.

3. WHAT FOR ACCREDITATION?

Till 1990 most of the hospitals, nursing homes are depending on cash paid patients. In olden days 90% of patients were paying hospital bills from their pockets and 10% of patients were referred by the big companies or insurance companies for cashless treatment as one of the staff welfare measures.

But in recent years it has been changed and cash paid patients have come down to 50%. The hospitals are also facing heavy competition among themselves as the patients are choosing their consultants and hospitals based on the facilities, quality of treatment, standards and cost of treatment. Patients choice on hospitals is on three factors;

i. Emergency: If any one met with an accident or falls on the road his first and immediate choice is to admit himself in the hospital which is very near to the accident spot. In this case there is no thinking, no option no choice except to admit in the near by hospital for first aid or treatment as delay may leads to serious health problems.

ii. Convenience: This is the second factor which helps patients to take decision regarding the choice of hospital. Locality where he lives and the hospital situated in that particular locality, transportation, facilities available, etc. will be the points for consideration of selecting a hospital.

iii. Loyalty: Loyalty is the most important factor and all the Health care providers should develop more this kind of patients. The patient will choose particular hospital for treatment irrespective of the distance, traffic and locality and cost.

Wherever he stays he goes to particular hospital even for small ailments or investigations, etc, as he is so loyal to that particular hospital. He is loyal because of his past experiences and he is very much satisfied with the facilities, treatment, respect and cost.

With the recent developments in the healthcare industries and government policies, the patient who come for hospital for treatment can be divided into the following categories:

i. Direct cash paid patients
ii. Patients referred by the companies, public sector undertakings on credit basis.
iii. Mediclaim patients where patients will settle the bills and claim reimbursement
iv. Insurance patients (TPAs) cashless treatment
v. CGHS scheme
vi. Medical tourism patients
vii. Government scheme patients (Arogyasree, Kalaigner scheme, etc.).

Since there is no rules and regulations or license to start a hospital, patients are choosing hospitals based on the facilities and professional expertise. Now QCI has constituted a separate board (NABH) for giving accreditation to the hospitals based on their standards. In near future, the patients referred by public sector undertakings, third party administrators (TPA) insurance companies, medical tourism patients may be insisted to admit for treatment in accreditated hospitals only. Since 50–60% of patients are either company referred patients or insurance patients in any multi speciality hospital the accreditation will become a mandatory for any hospital to face the competition.

Accreditation results in high quality of care and patients safety, patients or customer satisfaction is regularly evaluated. It raises community confidence in the services provided by the hospital. It also provides opportunity to the hospital to bench mark with the best.

4. HOW TO APPLY FOR ACCREDITATION?

Any multispecialty hospital or nursing home can apply to the Board of NABH for accreditation through the help of consultancy services or well trained in-house coordinators. The application can be downloaded from the Internet Website www.qci.org/nabh or it can be collected from the consultancy services.

Duly filled application has to be submitted along with necessary documents and fees. The application fees will be depending on number of beds. The local cheque (Delhi) or demand draft should be drawn in favor of Quality Council of India, payable at Delhi. The accreditation once granted will be valid for 3 years after which hospitals may apply for renewal as per NABH policy.

5. TIME LIMIT

There is no time limit for applying for accreditation. Any hospital when the systems are well defined and implemented it can apply for accreditation. Along with the application should be submitted pre-assessment tool. Auditng will be done by the Board and after rectification of deficiencies, if any, mentioned in the audit report, the members will do final assessment. If the audit team is satisfied with the standards of the Hospital the Board will issue an Accreditation certificate.

6. VALIDITY

The validity of certificate is for three years after completion of 3 years the hospital has to apply for its renewal as per rules and regulations of NABH.

7. WHO ARE ALL INVOLVED IN ACCREDITATION PROCESS?

The NABH audit is not a regular audit like bank audit or company audits where certain group of employees are involved. In NABH audit house keeping boy to CEO of the hospital is involved. Each and every category of employee working in hospital should be thorough in systems, hospital policies, procedures, scope of services, etc. Any staff in any department can be questioned by the audit team. Questions will be based on the subject or scope of service with which they deal. Ward boys, ayahs, para medical staff will be questioned by the audit team regarding disposal of biomedical wastage, vision and mission statement, services available in the hospital, HR policies, etc.

They expect the patient rights, hospital infection control methods, scope of service of the ward or department, etc. from the nursing staff.

The responsibility of top management is to keep and maintain all agreements, MOUs, licenses, certificates, etc. and follow the policies and procedures of the hospital.

8. WHO CAN APPLY FOR ACCREDITATION?

i. Multispeciality hospitals
   a. Trust hospitals
   b. Corporate hospitals
   c. Government hospitals

ii. Blood banks

iii. Nursing homes and small healthcare providers

iv. Wellness centers
   a. Gymnasiums centers
   b. Skin care center
   c. Cosmetic care centers
   d. Fitness centers
   e. Executive health check-up centers

v. Oral substitution therapy (OST) center (Narcoanalysis center) (Oral substitution therapy with buprenorphine)

vi. Medical laboratory program

vii. Medical imaging services
   a. X-ray units
   b. CT scan
   c. MRI scan
   d. Nuclear scan
   e. PET scan centers

viii. Ayush hospitals
   a. Ayurveda hospitals
   b. Homeopathy hospitals
   c. Unani hospitals
   d. Siddha hospitals
   e. Yoga and naturopathy hospitals.

9. APPLICATION FOR ACCREDITATION

The hospital shall apply to NABH in the prescribed application form. The application shall be accompanied with the following:
- Prescribed application fee as detailed in the application form
- Signed copy of 'Terms and Conditions for Maintaining NABH Accreditation' available free on the web-site
- Filled in self assessment toolkit, available free on the web-site
- Quality/hospital manual/apex manual (as per NABH standards) and other NABH relevant documents, i.e different policies and procedures of the hospital.

The applicant hospital must apply for all its facilities and services being rendered from the specific location.

10. SCRUTINY OF APPLICATION

NABH secretariat receives the application form and after scrutiny of application for its completeness in all respect, acknowledgement letter for the application shall be issued to the hospital with a unique reference number. The hospital shall be required to quote this reference number in all future correspondence with NABH.

11. PREASSESSMENT

NABH appoints a principle assessor/assessment team who is responsible for pre assessment of healthcare organization. NABH forwards the application form, documents, procedures, self assessment toolkit to the principle assessor/ assessment team.

12. OBJECTIVE OF PREASSESSMENT

- Check the preparedness of the hospital for final assessment
- Review the scope of accreditation and ascertain the requirement of the number of assessors and the duration of the accreditation
- Review of the documentation system of the hospital
- Explain the methodology to be adopted for assessment.

The Principle assessor shall submit a preassessment report in the format specified in the document 'preassessment guidelines and forms'. Copy of the report is handed over to the organization after the assessment and original sent to NABH Secretariat.

The hospital shall be required to pay the requisite Annual fee before the final assessment.

13. FINAL ASSESSMENT

The hospital is required to take necessary corrective action to the non-conformities pointed out during the preassessment. The final assessment involves comprehensive review of hospital functions and services. NABH shall appoint an assessment team. The team shall include principle assessor (already appointed) and the assessors. The total number of assessors appointed shall depend on the number of beds and services provided. The date of final assessment shall be agreed upon by the hospital management and assessors. Assessment shall be conducted on hospital's department and service.

Based on the assessment by the assessors, the assessment report is prepared by the principle assessor in a format prescribed by NABH.

The details of nonconformity (NC's) observed during the assessment are handed over to the hospital by the Principle assessor and detailed assessment report is sent to NABH.

14. SCRUTINY OF ASSESSMENT REPORT

NABH shall examine the assessment report. The report is taken to the accreditation committee. Depending on the score and compliance to standard would decided the award of accreditation or otherwise as per details given below.

i. Preaccreditation entry level: Conditions for qualifying to this award are as below:
   - All the regulatory legal requirements should be fully met
   - No individual standards should have more than one zeros
   - The average score for individual standard must not be less than 5
   - The average score for individual chapter must be more than 5
   - The overall average score for all standards must exceed 5.

   The validity period for pre-accreditation entry level stage is from a minimum 6 months to a maximum of 18 months. It means that a hospital placed under this award cannot apply for assessment before 6 months.

ii. Reaccreditation progressive level: Conditions for qualifying to this award are as below:
   - All the regulatory legal requirements should be fully met.
   - The average score for individual standard must not be less than 5
   - The average score for individual chapter must be more than 5
   - The overall average score for all standards must exceed 5.

   The validity period for reaccreditation progressive level stage is from a minimum 3 months to a maximum of 12 months. It means that a hospital placed under this award cannot apply for assessment before 3 months.

iii. Accredited: Conditions for qualifying for accreditation are as below:
   - All the regulatory legal requirements should be fully met.
   - No individual standard should have more than one zero to qualify
   - The average score for individual standards must not be less than 5
   - The average score for individual chapter must not be less than 7
   - The overall average score for all standards must exceed 7.

   The validity period for accreditation is 3 years subject to terms and conditions.

Note: The awards are only valid till the next assessment or until that last date of validity, whichever is earlier. Awards *cannot* be renewed. Depending upon the progress, the organization is eligible to get either a preaccreditation entry level award, preaccreditation progressive level award or accredited. If the organization under the stage of preaccreditation entry level and preaccreditation progressive level does not show any improvement during the next assessment they should be encouraged to apply afresh.

15. ISSUE OF ACCREDITATION CERTIFICATE

NABH shall issue an accreditation certificate to the hospital with a validity of three years. The certificate has a unique number and date of validity. The certificate is accompanied by scope of accreditation.

The applicant hospital must make all payment due to NABH, before the issue of certificate.

All decision taken by NABH regarding grant of accreditation shall be open to appeal by the hospitals, to chairman NABH.

16. SURVEILLANCE AND REASSESSMENT

Accreditation to a hospital shall be valid for a period of three years. NABH conducts one surveillance of the accredited hospitals in one accreditation cycle of three years. The surveillance visit will be planned during the 2nd year, i.e. after 18 months of accreditation.

The hospitals may apply for renewal of accreditation at least six months before the expiry of validity of accreditation for which reassessment shall be conducted.

The NABH may call for un-announced visit, based on any concern or any serious incident reported upon by an individual or organization or media.

CHAPTERS IN NABH

Chapter 1	Access, Assessment and Continuity of Care (AAC)
Chapter 2	Care of Patients (COP)
Chapter 3	Management of Medication (MOM)
Chapter 4	Patient Rights and Education (PRE)
Chapter 5	Hospital Infection Control (HIC)
Chapter 6	Continuous Quality Improvement (CQI)
Chapter 7	Responsibility of Management (ROM)
Chapter 8	Facility Management and Safety (FMS)
Chapter 9	Human Resource Manager (HRM)
Chapter 10	Information Management System (IMS)

Out of 10 chapters first 5 chapters are medical chapters and remaining 5 chapters are administrative chapters.

Details of Chapters, Standards and Subjects

S.Number	Chapter	Standard	Subjects
1.	AAC	14	86
2.	COP	20	136
3.	MOM	13	73
4.	PRE	7	46
5.	HIC	9	51
6.	CQI	8	57
7.	ROM	6	38
8.	FMS	8	54
9.	HRM	10	52
10.	IMS	7	43
	Total	102	636

NABH POLICIES CHAPTERWISE

Chapter 1—Access, Assessment and Continuity of Care

- Policies on laboratory service
- Laboratory quality assurance manual
- Laboratory safety program
- Policy and procedure for discharge of patients
- Policy on admission of patients
- Policy on assessment and reassessment of patients
- Policy on assessment of OPD patients
- Policy and procedure guiding transfer/referral of stable/unstable patients to other organizations.
- Policy on continuum of care
- Policy on in-house transfer of patients
- Policy for leave against medical advise (LAMA)
- Policy on reduction of barriers and information of resources
- Policy on right to access of care
- Policy and procedure on nonavailability of bed
- Policy on clinical assessment of patient—IP/OP/emergency, preventive aspection, plan of care
- Policy on regular reassessment of patients with detailed treatment plan.

Chapter 2—Care of Patients

- Policy on use of blood and blood products
- Policy for blood availability for emergency use
- Policy on documentation of continuous patient care, multidisciplinary approach with defined roles and responsibilities; for example, nurses/ technician/duty doctor/register
- Policy on care of patients
- Policy addressing emergency patients
- Policy for referral of patients to other specialties
- Policy on care of vulnerable group of patients
- Policy on end of life care
- Policy on preventing fall
- Policy on patient identification
- Policy to prevent child, abduction and abuse
- Policy for ambulance services
- Policy on surgical care of patients
- Policy on transferring out patients from recovery room to ICUs or wards
- Policy for admission and discharge criteria's for ICUs
- Procedure for prevention of adverse events like wrong site, wrong patient and wrong surgery

- Policy for triage of patients
- Policy on cardiopulmonary resuscitation
- Policy on management of poster operative pain
- Policy on radiology services
- Radiation safety program
- Radiation quality assurance manual
- Policy on surgical care of patients
- Policy for use of sedation
- Policy on use of restraints
- Policy for administration and monitored anesthesia care
- Hazardous material management plan
- Policy on rehabilitative services
- Policy guiding nutritional and reassessment
- Policy on research activities.

Chapter 3—Management of Medication

- Policy for protecting medications from loss or theft
- Policy for emergency/crash cart
- Policy for medications not listed in the formulary
- Policy for prescription of medications
- Policy for storage of medications
- Policy for obtaining medications when pharmacy is closed
- Policy for medication recall
- Policy on discarding opened medication
- Policy on drug formulary
- Policy for medications not listed in the formulary
- Policy on storage of medication
- Policy for medication administration
- Policy on adverse reaction
- Policy on medication error
- Policy for medication administration
- Policy on verbal orders
- Policy for self medication
- Policy on narcotic drugs
- Handling of cytotoxic drugs
- Patient education on medication
- Policy on high-risk medication
- Policy and procedure on procurement of implantable prosthesis
- Medical gas safety program.

Chapter 4—Patient Rights and Education

- Policy and procedure on informed consent
- List of procedures for which informed consent and high-risk consent is required
- Policy on visitor/patient feedback
- Policy on patient and family education
- Pricing policy
- Policy on patient and family rights
- Policy on staff training on the services offered various hospital policies
- Policy on services offered by the organization.

Chapter 5—Hospital Infection Control

- Policy on infection control program
- Policy on high risk areas in the hospital
- Policy on standard precautions
- Policy on kitchen sanitation and food handling
- Policy on isolation
- Policy on investigation on outbreak
- Policy on personnel protective equipment
- Policy on handling of linen
- Cleaning and disinfections
- Policy on handling of dead bodies
- Policy on notifiable infectious diseases
- Policy on hospital waste management
- Policy on hand hygiene
- Policy on cssd recall procedure
- Antibiotic guidelines
- Policy on surveillance including high risk area's
- Policy on employee health and vaccination
- Outline of procedure for sterilization activities
- Policy on reuse of device.

Chapter 6—Continuous Quality Improvement

- Quality assurance program
- Policy on sentinel events
- Policy on medical audits
- Policy on quality indicators.

Chapter 7—Responsibility of Management

- Policy for organization social responsibility.

Chapter 8—Facility Management and Safety

- Safety manual
- Policy on disaster management
- Evacuation plan
- Policy on emergency evacuation plan
- Policy on safety committee
- Smoking policy
- Policy on facility management and safety
- Policy on patient safety
- Policy on visitors
- Policy on patient valuables
- Hazardous material management plan
- Policy on operational and maintenances plan including preventive maintenance.

Chapter 9—Human Resource Management

- Policy on HR management and manpower planning
- Recruitment
- Performance appraisal
- Safety on staff
- Training matrix
- Clinical staff credentials
- Job description and KRA's
- Disciplinary policy
- Grievance handling policy
- Policy on responsibilities of management organization chart, governance issues, legal issues, CSR, roles and responsibilities
- Credentialing and privileging of staff
- Policy on health check of employees.

Chapter 10—Information Management system

- Contents of medical records
- Confidentiality and privacy policy
- Authorization of making entries in medical records
- Policy of safeguarding data record against loss, destruction and tampering
- Policy on disposal of medical records
- Order of filing medical records (checklist)
- Policy on access of medical records
- Policy on storage of medical records
- Policy on medicolegal cases
- Policy on request of medical records by patient and attendant

- Confidentiality and privacy policy
- Authorization of making entries in HIS
- Information requirements of the organization
- Procedure for timely and accurate dissemination of data
- Policy on technology acquisition
- Procedure to meet information needs.

IMPORTANT ASPECTS FOR ACCREDITATION

System is nothing but a way of organizing things according to the policies and principles of organization in a sequence.

There are:

a. Natural system
b. Mechanical system
c. Administrative system

a. We have no role in natural system except to observe or to maintain, examples for natural system is like solar system, body system, digestive system, etc.
b. Mechanical system are made by human beings. How xerox machine works, how X-ray machine works. How rocket flies in to the space. All these machines are designed and work on particular system after scientific experiments and proof.
c. Administrative system are created by the top management/administrators according to the polices and principles of the organization. It may differ from organization to organization.

Good systems are essential for the growth of the organization.

Systems should be (a) clear, (b) simple, and (c) transparent.

If a patient wants to give blood sample for test, first of all he should know where to give and whether blood will be drawn before or after making payment in the cash counter.

Secondly, the cash counter should available next to the billing section or billing staff will himself collect cash. The procedure should be simple and it should not be a complicated one.

Then system should be transparent and any one working in hospital should know the procedure of cash payment, like this entire system of hospital should be known to the staff, patients, attenders and it should be simple.

Good systems are like forming a road for smooth, comfortable and safe travel.

As per NABH norms there is no fixed systems for hospitals. But the system formed by the organization should be understandable, comfortable and safe to the patients and also to the staff working in departments of the hospital.

The important aspects for accreditation are as follows.

Documentation

Documentation is one of the important aspect for accreditation. The polices and procedures of the hospital should be documented properly. Documentation is nothing but recording or writing in a register or case-sheets what has done to the patient or what happened in the department in a fixed format.

NABH is particulars about two things:

1. What is being followed in the wards or departments should be documented
2. What is documented should be followed.

NABH is not concern about your notices and procedure and it does not have fixed formats that all the hospitals should follow the prescribed formats. But the polices and procedures of hospital should be clear, transparent and safe to the patients, staff and organization.

For each and every subject (635) in 102 standard of 10 chapters, the detailed policies and procedures of the hospital should be clearly mentioned and the same should be submitted to NABH. What is being followed only should be mentioned in documents should be followed strictly.

If the hospital does not have policies and systems for some of the subjects, it can be decided by the hospital authorities at the time of filling the documents.

Manuals

Preparation of manuals for each and every department in the hospital is very important.

1. Administrative department
2. Service department
   Electrical, pluming, air-conditioning, medical gases, carpenters, painting, etc.
3. Investigation departments
   Lab, X-ray, ECG, ultrasound, echo, cath lab, treadmill, CT scan, MRI scan, etc.
4. Inpatient wards
5. Operation theaters.

Manual of every department should have the following details:

1. Name of the department
2. Location of the department
3. Scope of service (Administration of department)
4. Staff details, equipment, furniture, resource management

5. Quality indicators
6. Department profile—staff hierarchy
7. Department policies
8. Vision and Mission statement of the organization.

In every ward the following registers has to be maintained:
1. Scope of service
2. Medicines stock registers
3. Narcotic drugs registers
4. Accident and incident registers
5. Key indicators registers
6. Resource management
7. Department polices
8. Department profile
9. Details of patients.

Administrative department:
1. Scope of services
2. Accident and incident registers
3. Key indicator register
4. Resource management
5. Department polices
6. Department profile.

Investigation department:
1. Scope of service
2. Accident and incident registers
3. Key indicator registers
4. Resource management
5. Department polices
6. Department profile
7. Details of patients.

Service departments:
1. Scope of service
2. Accident and incident registers
3. Complaint registers
4. Resource management
5. Department polices
6. Department profile.

In addition to this manuals, for entire hospital the following manuals has to be prepared.

1. Hospital infection control manual
2. Safety manual
3. Radiation safety manual
4. Laboratory QA manual
5. Laboratory safety manual
6. Hospital QA manual.

Mandatory training programs:

S.Number	*Nurses*	*Doctors*
1.	Induction program for new employees	Induction program
2.	Job responsibility	Job responsibility
3.	Awareness about appraisal at the time of induction	Awareness of grievance
4.	Awareness about disciplinary procedure	Training for disciplinary procedure
5.	Awareness about grievance	Training for non availability of beds
6.	Risk within the hospital environment, ex. fire, Non firc emergencies, needle stick injury	Training for ACLS
7.	Internal department training program	Training for CPR
8.	Employee rights and responsibilities	Hand hygiene
9.	New equipment introduced	Infection control protocol
10.	Scope of service	Fire emergency
11.	Non availability of beds	Safety education program
12.	BLS/ACLS training	Disaster management
13.	CPR Training	
14.	Admission and discharge criteria for ICU	
15.	How to handle vulnerable patient and define	
16.	Staff should train how to take care of pediatric patients	

17. Training for restrain techniques
18. Training for end of life care
19. How to administer chemotherapy drugs
20. Training about patient rights and responsibilities
21. Training for hand washing techniques
22. Training for infection control program
23. Training for biomedical waste practices (color codes and PPE's)
24. Staff should be trained for their roles and responsibilities for fire emergency
25. Staff should be trained for hospital disaster management plan
26. Staff should be trained for handling the hazardous materials
    Staff should be trained for safety Education program.

To continue to maintain the quality of service and standards even after getting NABH accreditation certificate the management should create three powerful teams with an efficient staff:

They are:
- Quality assurance team
- Hospital infection control team
- Audit team.

Quality assurance team mainly concentrate on quality of services, safety of patients attendants and staff, performance of key indicators, etc.

Hospital infection control team will concentrate on periodical surveillance of all high-risk areas, giving training to ward staff in hand washing technique, controlling and prevention of hospital associated infection, monitoring antibiotic policy and its implementation, any outbreaks in the hospital, etc.

Audit team is mainly to audit the departments in the hospital and give report to the management through quality assurance team. There are three types of auditing:
- Auditing of documents
- Auditing of systems
- Auditing of materials (inventory)

Staff in all three team should have good traits to get good results to the hospital.

- They should be polite and soft spoken.
- They should have thorough knowledge about their field of operation.
- They should be friendly with the costaff and help them in training and implementing the various standards of NABH.
- The team member should be permanent and there should not be frequent changes of members to maintain the uniform systems.
- There should be a checklist and prescribed procedure for each team to help the new members.
- The system and procedures suggested by the team members should be as per the norms of NABH and they should not be individual based systems and procedures.
- If any suggestions for better services to the patient by any member of the team should be implemented through the approval of the management.
- Periodical reports should be submitted by the team members to the top management.
- The top management should maintain the activity of the team member.
- The team members should be unbiased while performing their duties.

CHAPTER 32

Licenses and Acts Applicable to Hospitals

ACTS APPLICABLE

Various Acts that are applicable for establishing, running the hospital are as follows:

1. Charitable and Religious Trusts Act, 1920 (if the hospital is a trust hospital)
2. Consumer Protection Act, 1986
3. Contract Act, 1982
4. Customs Act, 1962
5. Drugs and Cosmetics Act, 1940
6. Electricity Rules, 1956
7. Employees Provident Fund, 1956
8. ESI ACT, 1948 (only for Canteen Staff)
9. Income Tax Act, 1961
10. National Holidays under shops Act
11. Indian Trade Unions Act, 1926
12. Industrial Dispute Act, 1947
13. Maternity Benefit Act, 1961
14. MTP Act, 1971
15. Minimum Wages Act, 1948
16. Payments of Wages Act, 1936
17. Payments of Gratuity Act, 1972
18. Pharmacy Act, 1948
19. Registration of Births and Deaths Act, 1969
20. Sales Tax Act
21. Insurance Act, 1938
22. Workers Compensation Act, 1923
23. Urban Land Act, 1976

24. PNDT Act, 1996
25. Companies Act (Applicable if the hospital is a corporate hospital).

LIST OF RENEWAL LICENCES

S.No.	*Licenses*	*Purpose*
1.	No objection certificate from the chief fire officer	for buildings
2.	Permit to operate lifts under the lifts act	for safety of the Lifts
3	Tamil Nadu Pollution Control Board (Biomedical waste management handling)	for disposal of Bio medical waste
4	PNDT-License as per act, 1996	License for pre-neonatal diagnostic facilities
5.	Corporation license for canteen	for running canteen in the premises
6.	License for blood bank	for running blood bank
7.	Transplantation of Human Organs Act,1994	1994 for organ transplant surgery
8.	No objection certificate from Tamilnadu	for disposal of sewage water pollution control board
9.	Narcotic and Psychotropic Substances Act	for administration of Narcotic and psychotropic drugs (on patient)
10.	Atomic energy regulatory board	for keeping and dealing with Isotopes for nuclear scan department/pet scan
11.	Radiation protection certificates in respect of all imaging department from AERB	Drug license for sale of medicines
12.	Drug license	National 1956 (DNB) Board of Examinations
13.	Indian Medical Council Act and code for running diploma courses in medical ethics,	As per State Government rules
14.	Registration for hospital (local municipality/corporation	if the cylinder capacity is more 1000 lts
15.	Chief control of explosive license for storage of liquid oxygen	

LIST OF PERMANENT LICENSES

Building permit (from the municipality)

1. Income Tax Pan Number.
2. Sales Tax Registration Certificate (Tin No).
3. Service Tax Registration Number (STC).
4. Tax deducted at source (Tan Number).
5. Vehicle registration certificate for all the vehicles.

Any other Acts and licenses are applicable as per the local bodies or the state government regulation where the hospital is located.

Bibliography

1. Hand book of Hospital Personnel management By Goyal.
2. Finance management By Chandra.
3. Standard operating Procedures for hospital By Arun K Agarwal.
4. Definition of Consumer Protection Act By Dr Gurbax Singh.
5. Australian Guide for blood donation.
6. www.medindia.net/cpa.
7. wikipedea.org/wiki/Medical – Ethics.
8. www.indianarmy.nic.in.
9. QCI-NABH standards.
10. www.leadership-and-motivation-trainining.com/motivational factors.
11. www.Ahrq.gov.
12. Blood transfusion therapy –aa/bb.
13. The clinical use of blood——WHO, Geneva.
14. Mci india.org.
15. Medicalgases-enotes.com.
16. e-how.com.
17. irishhealth.com.
18. Bhargava Associates.
19. Patientsafety.co.in.
20. Rayrichardson.blogspot.in.
21. Creating an Inspiring work Environment (Motivational techniques). By Scott Jeffry.
22. Hospmgt.tripod.com/committees.
23. Indmedia/com.
24. In answers.yahoo.com.
25. Art-ofopatient.com.
26. A great practical guide to clinical medical ethics for health professionals.
27. A practical approach to Ethical Decisions in Clinical Medicine-Sixth edition.

28. Berger C, Calabrese R. "Some Explanations in Initial Interaction and Beyond: Toward a Developmental Theory of Interpersonal Communication". Human Communication Research. 1975;1:99-112.
29. Wanzer MB, Booth-Butterfiled M, Gruber K. "Perceptions of Health Care Providers' Communication: Relationships between Patient-Centered Communication and Satisfaction". Health Communication, 2004;16(3):363-84.
30. Parasuraman A, Berry LL, Zeithaml VA. "Refinement and Reassessment of the SERVQUAL Scale". Journal of Retailing. 1991;67:420-50.
31. Strawderman L, Koubek R. "Quality and Usability in a Student Health Clinic". International Journal of Health Care Quality Assurance. 2006;19:225-36.

Index